Probiotics in Mental Health

Probiotics in Mental Health

Editors

Colin R Martin

Faculty of Society and Health
Buckinghamshire New University, Uxbridge, UK

Derek Larkin

Department of Psychology
Edge Hill University, Ormskirk, Lancashire, UK

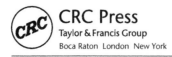

CRC Press is an imprint of the
Taylor & Francis Group, an **informa** business

A SCIENCE PUBLISHERS BOOK

Cover credit: Illustrations taken from Chapter 4.

CRC Press
Taylor & Francis Group
6000 Broken Sound Parkway NW, Suite 300
Boca Raton, FL 33487-2742

First issued in paperback 2021

© 2018 by Taylor & Francis Group, LLC
CRC Press is an imprint of Taylor & Francis Group, an Informa business

No claim to original U.S. Government works

Version Date: 20171214

ISBN-13: 978-0-367-78115-6 (pbk)
ISBN-13: 978-1-4665-7356-7 (hbk)

Library of Congress Cataloging-in-Publication Data

Names: Martin, Colin R., 1964- editor.
Title: Probiotics in mental health / editors, Colin R. Martin and Derek
  Larkin.
Description: Boca Raton, FL : CRC Press, Taylor & Francis Group, [2018] | "A
  science publishers book." | Includes bibliographical references and index.
Identifiers: LCCN 2017057525 | ISBN 9781466573567 (hardback : alk. paper)
Subjects: LCSH: Mental illness--Treatment. | Probiotics--Therapeutic use. |
  Gastrointestinal system--Microbiology.
Classification: LCC RC480 .P69 2018 | DDC 616.89/1--dc23
LC record available at https://lccn.loc.gov/2017057525

Visit the Taylor & Francis Web site at
http://www.taylorandfrancis.com

and the CRC Press Web site at
http://www.crcpress.com

Dedication

Colin R Martin—I would like to dedicate this book to my beautiful daughter Caragh Brien, in her third year at medical school and of whom I am so proud.

Derek Larkin—I would like to dedicate this book to my partner Karen Ann Nicklin whose love and guidance has been impressive. She is my best friend, staunch ally, most able critic, and my role model. For my part I would also like to dedicate this book to my in-laws (Iris, Norman and Nigel) simply because they bring laughter in to my life—Thank you.

Acknowledgements

The Editors would like to acknowledge each contributor in turn, this book would not have been accomplished without their hard work, professionalism and dedication. We are also grateful to our friends and colleagues who have provided us with extensive personal and professional guidance.

Foreword

The recent interest in the relationship between the gut and well-being has been an intriguing development within, till recently, the biosciences. Interestingly, from that perspective, the focus has been largely in the area of physical well-being. However, this is changing as the relationship between the gut and the brain, which, though undeniably complex, begins to present compelling evidence for a significant relationship with mental health. This is important as it allows us to consider the emergence of some mental health problems in a novel way and allows us to contrast this new evidence with existing models, irrespective of whether they be medical, psychosocial or genetic models. A fundamentally exciting position also presents itself with this emerging evidence base of the gut–brain axis for those of us working within the clinical sphere, and that is the potential for interventions that may be effective and also benign, particularly when one considers the side-effect profile that is associated with many of the pharmacological interventions used within the mental health field. The area of probiotics and mental health thus represents a comparatively new field, a science in its infancy and yet, even at this early stage of evolution, finding novel and robust outcomes with significant implications for potential intervention strategies.

Reflecting on the potential role of probiotics to help with mental health problems provides a seductive context for a number of potential 'thought experiments'. It is thus plausible to consider in a scientific and robust way, the relationship between the gut–brain axis and the manifestation of significant mental health problems within an aetiological perspective. Thus, if we are able to establish a relationship between for example, the gut–brain axis and depression, what does this mean in terms of diagnosis, course and outcome? Given the complexity of diagnostic systems used within clinical psychiatry, could this be considered a unitary model of depression, embracing all accounts of diagnosed depression, or could this be the context to define a new type of depression, with a different cause, treatment and outcome, to say, for example, an endogenous depression defined within an aetiological model of low 5-Hydroxytriptamine (serotonin) levels, which would of course would likely define a pharmacological intervention approach, usually with selective serotonin reuptake inhibitors (SSRI's). Considering just this single premise then, a constellation of pertinent factors begins to emerge regarding, diagnosis, course and prognosis.

The above presents just one potential possibility that the area of probiotics and mental health brings in facilitating innovation and renewal in the provision of evidence-based mental health care. A second exciting possibility is that through effective patient education in the link between the gut–brain axis and mental health problems, in the example of where the relationship is proven within the context of an individual patient, the scope for considering the role of the patient in their own recovery and mastery of their mental health challenges is legion. In many respects, the patient may be encouraged to take a far more dynamic role in their mental health care through education regarding the gut–brain axis and how they can influence this by dietary and probiotic intervention. Circumstances such as these then, may provide opportunities to influence individual mental health and well-being and by engagement, critical aspects of experience which are related to good mental health, such as increased self-efficacy. The current maturity of the probiotics and mental health field is currently at a stage of infancy; thus, the above possibilities are simply that at the present time, possibilities for future consideration. However, as the field develops, these kinds of questions raised will require answers and, the development of mechanisms where they can be embraced within the context of service delivery, under the rubric that mechanisms of action can be established for specific mental health presentations.

Reflecting on my own area of interest in clinical psychiatry, specifically forensic psychotherapy, it is most notable when thinking about the contents of this new book that psychoanalytic psychotherapy and the approaches and theoretical models that underpin it, consider food as metaphor within the psychodynamic space. If one was to consider, from a psychoanalytic perspective, an early care-giving environment devoid of empathy and love, both passive and distancing from the mother object, food may become the substitute symbolic representation to fill this vacuum. It is striking that within the realm of psychoanalysis, the role of food within the therapeutic encounter has been of relevance, even back to Freud's early and seminal work. It should therefore not be too surprising that as science evolves to understand at a deeper and more sophisticated level, multi-modal mechanisms that influence mental health, that robust notions of classical thinking about significant psychological disturbance, can be renewed and enhanced by developments such as this area of work in probiotics.

Colin Martin and Derek Larkin have done an excellent job bringing together clinicians and researchers within the probiotics and mental health fields to present a compelling and evidence-based discourse on the role of probiotics in understanding and the potential role of treatment in the presentations defined by significant mental health concerns. Professor Martin and Dr Larkin acknowledge the current status of the probiotics and mental health evidence base as an emerging area and the chapter on research methodologies is particularly appealing in this regard. Most of the chapters are presented by a particular mental health diagnosis, which makes the text accessible for those of us more familiar within clearly defined diagnostic boundaries.

This book provides an up-to-date, engaging and compelling account of the potential role of probiotics in both understanding specific mental health presentations and highlighting the potential for novel interventions couched within plausible accounts of the gut–brain access. This book is thus consequently suitable for a broad range of readership with an interest in this interdisciplinary discourse.

Finally, I am optimistic that this book will 'raise the game' in terms of the conversation about the role of probiotics in relation to application and also, to foster the debate around, where the efficacy of these approaches can be shown and replicated, how best to incorporate such approaches within the clinical battery, to enhance patient choice, engagement and outcome.

Professor Gabriel Kirtchuk
Consultant psychiatrist in psychotherapy at West London Mental Health NHS Trust
and Fellow of the British Psychoanalytical Society
London, UK

Preface

There has been an explosion of interest in the potential role of probiotics in relation to health, disease and homeostasis. The contemporary evidence base in relation to therapeutic promise continues to develop at an ever increasing rate as more studies find links between probiotics and disease/health status. Against this broad picture of probiotics and health, a more specific area of interest has emerged with respect to the relationship between probiotics and mental health. The focus of this book is to examine in detail the evidence, mechanisms and therapeutic potential of the use of probiotics in a range of mental health conditions and diagnoses. This volume examines the role of probiotics with regard to established mental health conditions with an established pedigree of aetiology, diagnosis and prognosis such as depression and schizophrenia while also examining the therapeutic potential and mechanisms of probiotic action in more ambiguous and vexing diagnoses with a mental health component such as chronic fatigue syndrome. This book aims to give a comprehensive overview of the role of probiotics in mental health and mental well-being, summarising the contemporary evidence and examining some of the challenges of research and evidence-based practice in this exciting and dynamic area.

Colin R. Martin
Derek Larkin

Contents

Chapter 1

Introduction
Probiotics and Psychopathology

Derek Larkin[1],* and Colin R Martin[2]

INTRODUCTION

As you will read throughout the proceeding chapters Probiotics and Psychopathology are fascinating topics in their own right, but when combined they illustrate a complete and intriguing link between our gastrointestinal bacteria and the nervous system.

The concept that the gut and brain are intricately linked, and their interactions are to a large extent intuitive, are millennia old and are deeply rooted in our language (Mayer, 2011). Terms such as "heartache" and "gut wrenching" are more than mere metaphor, we feel the ache of love and loss in our chest and abdomen. We experience an orchestral repertoire of emotions in our hearts and stomachs in the form of muscle tightness, or increased heart rate, or abnormal contractions of the stomach— the emotional areas of our brain are inextricably connected to pain regions. The interlink or crosstalk between the gut and brain has revealed a complex bidirectional communication system that appears to help not only maintain gastrointestinal homoeostasis, but is also likely to affect our mental and emotional wellbeing (Emery and Coan, 2010).

The pathway linking the nervous system and the digestive system was first discovered in the nineteenth century and was subsequently labelled the enteric nervous system (Furness, 2008; Furness and Costa, 1987). The enteric nervous system is considered the third branch of the autonomic nervous system, and has been termed the 'second brain' (Gershon, 1998; Mayer, 2011). It shares a similar size, complexity, and similarity in neurotransmitter, and signalling molecules with the brain (Gershon, 1998; Mayer, 2011).

---

[1] Edge Hill University, St Helens Road, Ormsirk, Lancashire, L39 4QP.
[2] Faculty of Society and Health, Buckinghamshire New University, Uxbridge Campus, 106 Oxford Road, Uxbridge, Middlesex, UB8 1NA, UK.
* Corresponding author

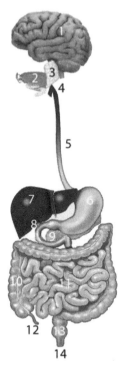

Figure 1 1. Human Brain, 2. Tongue, 3. Saliva Glands, 4. Pharynx, 5. Oesophagus, 6. Stomach, 7. Liver, 8. Gallbladder, 9. Pancreas, 10. Large Intestines, 11. Small Intestines, 12. Appendix, 13. Rectum, 14. Anus Figure adapted from https://www.britannica.com/science/human-digestive-system. (© 2003 encyclopedia Britannica, Inc.)

The interaction between the brain and the digestive system and their relationship with health and disease has been recognised for many centuries, and studied by ancient cultures, and in modern times by psychologists and physiologists (Mayer and Brunnhuber, 2012). There has been a long-term appreciation that there is an association between several chronic gastrointestinal tract disorders and psychiatric symptoms. While different theories have been proposed, the direction of causality and the precise nature of the underlying pathophysiology remains incomplete (Mayer and Brunnhuber, 2012). Nevertheless, recent scientific advances in the emerging fields of 'enteric neuroscience' and 'emotional neuroscience' have been instrumental in understanding the bidirectional brain–gut interaction (Mayer, 2011; Mayer and Brunnhuber, 2012). According to Mayer and Brunnhuber (2012) many clinicians continue to adhere to Cartesian dualism when treating patients with chronic gastrointestinal disorders. This idea implies that many gastroenterologists refrain from acknowledging the significant role played by the central nervous system in many disorders, which may include inflammatory bowel disease, or chronic oesophageal disorder. They dismiss psychological and psychiatric factors in the manifestation and maintenance of the disease process as neurotic hysterical behaviours which are only peripheral to the condition. In contrast psychologists and psychiatrics tend to embrace the concept of somatization; the manifestation of psychological distress by the presentation of bodily symptoms (Rhee et al., 2009). There is however still a rudimentary understanding of the involvement of the enteric microbiota including the commensal bacterial flora present within the gastrointestinal tract, which is part of the normal function of the gut. Consequently, the role of the enteric microbiota in the bidirectional gut–brain interaction in relation to general health and disease has received little empirical enquiry (Rhee et al., 2009).

The human digestive system is thought to be home to 400–1000 different species of bacteria, which make up an intricate network of cohabiting organisms (Mazmanian et al., 2008). The enteric microbiota can influence gut homeostasis by the regulation of bowel motility, modulation of intestinal pain, immune response, and nutrient processing (Ait-Belgnaoui et al., 2006; Husebye et al., 2001; Rhee et al., 2005; Rhee et al., 2009). There is a growing school of thought and mounting empirical research that is increasingly examining the symbiotic relationship between the enteric microbiota and their human host. This school of thought is driving afresh, an understanding of the importance of the two systems in maintaining homeostasis health (Turnbaugh et al., 2007).

Tremendous progress has been made in characterizing the bidirectional interactions between the central nervous system, the enteric nervous system, and the gastrointestinal tract. There is growing evidence of the fact that gut microbiota has a powerful influence on gut–brain interactions. There is also growing evidence of gut microbiota influence and development of emotional behaviour as well as stress and pain modulation, and brain neurotransmitter systems (Mayer et al., 2015). Pre- and probiotics have been used to modulate gut microbiota to measure multiple biological systems that may ultimately influence behaviour via the autonomic nervous system, but there is limited information as to how these findings may translate to human health or the disease state, involving the brain or the gut–brain axis. But evidence is mounting which suggests the symbiotic bidirectional brain–gut relationship has other important features that relate to not only our physical well-being but also our psychopathology, outlined in each of the preceding chapters.

Probiotics

The word 'probiotics' was derived many thousands of years after it was known that certain food supplements had beneficial effects. The etymology of 'probiotic' is derived from the meaning 'for life' in Greek, but has had several meanings over the years. Probiotic is in essence described as a substance that is secreted by one microorganism which stimulates the growth of another (Fuller, 2012). However, a more complete definition that was commonly accepted was first used by Parker (1974), organisms and substances which contribute to intestinal microbiota balance. Nevertheless, this definition was thought to have included all microbial substances including 'antibiotics' as such Fuller (1989) redefined probiotics as 'the live microbial feed supplement which beneficially affects the host animal by improving its intestinal microbial balance', thus emphasising the viability of the supplement. The WHO define probiotics as 'a live organism', which when administered in adequate amounts, confer health benefits on the host (Schlundt, 2001).

The exact point in history in which the manufacture of fermented milks was first used is almost impossible to establish, but it has been estimated that the date could be as old as 10,000 years ago, as life moved from just gathering food to food production, and the domestication and animal husbandry of cows, sheep, goats, buffalo and camel (Pederson, 1971; Tamime, 2002). Agricultural records appear to suggest that the Sumerians, Babylonians, Pharos and Indian cultures may have been among the first to cultivate this complex process (Pederson, 1971). The consumption of fermented milk is now common place in many parts of the world, and across all cultures.

Yoghurts and sour milk were the first to come under scientific scrutiny. Work conducted at the Pasteur Institute in Paris were among the first to explore a long-regarded notion that microflora of the lower gut had adverse and beneficial effects on the health of the human adult (Fuller, 2012). Early pioneers advocated the use of milk fermented with the single strain of *Lactobacillus* (a genus of Gram positive, facultative anaerobic microaerophilic, rod shaped, non-spore forming bacteria) still used today and remains one of the most common used probiotic organisms—in which it converts sugars to lactic acid.

The Nobel Prize recipient Eli Metchnikoff working at the Pasteur Institute during the early part of the 1900s stated "The dependence of the intestinal microbes on food makes it possible to adopt measures to modify the flora in our bodies and to replace harmful microbes with useful microbes" (Metchnikoff, 1907). Around the same time a French paediatrician called Henry Tissier, noticed that children with diarrhoea had low numbers of a particular bacteria within their stool samples, one that was plentiful in healthy children. The bacteria had a distinctive Y-shaped morphology or 'bifid'. He suggested that bacteria from the gut of healthy children could be administered to those with diarrhoea to help restore healthy gut flora (Tissier, 1906; as cited in Schlundt, 2001). The work of Metchnikoff and Tissier was subsequently commercially exploited however, not all results were positive, and many observations that at first glance appeared scientifically stable, were however shown to be unproven or anecdotal. Probiotic research subsequently fell out of favour but, in the last 30 years' research concerning probiotics has found a resurgence.

Lactobacillus and *Bifidobacterium* are the most commercially exploited probiotic microorganisms, used in numerous food products available to consumers. Under normal circumstances (when the host microbiota has not been compromised as a consequence of disease) the gastrointestinal tract is home to some 400-obligate anaerobic bacterial species (Schlundt, 2001; Tannock et al., 2000). Bacterial colonisation begins at birth; bacterial colonisation of the neonates' gastrointestinal tract begins during the birth process when the neonate comes into contact with maternal cervical and vaginal flora (Bezirtzoglou, 1997). Neonates delivered by caesarean section recieve their bacteria colonisation via contact with the environment. The colonisation of intestinal microflora has a number of beneficial roles, referred to as 'colonisation resistance' or the 'barrier effect' (Vollaard and Clasener, 1994). This is to say that intestinal flora would resist the recolonization of freshly ingested microorganisms which could include pathogens. As such it could be suggested that dietary manipulation of gut flora in order to increase the relative numbers of 'beneficial bacteria' could contribute to the well-being of the host (Schlundt, 2001).

Psychopathology

Psychopathology is the scientific study of mental disorders, and includes the scientific exploration in order to understand the underlying genetic, biological, psychological, and social causes, their development and their manifestations, and a study of the treatments.

Etymology of 'Psychopathology' has Greek meaning; psyche meaning 'soul', pathos meaning 'suffering', and logos is 'the study of'. In essence, therefore psychopathology means 'study of the suffering soul'. Psychologists and psychiatrists who specialise in mental health, diagnosis, and treatment of patients, use specific diagnostic criteria and symptomology found in the *Diagnostic and Statistical Manual of Mental Disorders*.

The *Diagnostic and Statistical Manual of Mental Disorders* (DSM) is currently in its fifth edition (American Psychiatric Association, 2013) having superseded the DSM-IV-TR (American Psychiatric Association, 2000) in May 2013. The DSM is the standard reference manual for assessment, and diagnosis of neuropsychiatric conditions. The first edition of the DSM evolved out of the international classification of diseases (ICD-6) in 1952. Its goal ever since has been to map knowledge about the brain and psychopathologies, and to guide clinical professionals on the diagnosis of mental health disorders. One of the guiding principles of the DSM is to evaluate knowledge and to stay abreast of the changing times and the developments in causes and diagnosis of neuropsychiatric conditions.

Probiotics, Mental Health, and Intestinal Microbiota

Reports suggest that there is a global mental health crisis which is increasingly seen as a consequence of modernisation, at least to some degree (Bested et al., 2013). It has been theorised that changes in socioeconomics, increasing demands for urbanization, alterations in dietary habits, sedentary behaviour, increasingly more time watching TV or interacting with computers, lack of adequate sunlight, erosion of real world (off-line) social support, and a disconnect from nature, are thought to be contributing factors to the prevalence of many health concerns (Bested et al., 2013; Colla et al., 2006; Hidaka, 2012; Logan and Selhub, 2012). Research groups around the globe are starting to explore the interaction of these influences and how they combine with other features of modern life that impose on mental health (Bested et al., 2013).

An area of research increasing in popularity involves neuropsychological consequences of modifications to gut microbiota (Dinan and Quigley, 2011). Logan and Katzman (2005); Logan et al. (2003) have argued the beneficial role of probiotics in the conditions of human fatigue and depressive disorders. They argue that mental health disorders are associated with low grade inflammation, oxidative stress, and the elevation of inflammatory cytokines. Studies have shown that mood disorders and fatigue could be induced by systematic administration of lipopolysaccharide endotoxin (Dinan and Quigley, 2011). Studies have also shown that probiotics could influence systemic cytokines, oxidative stress, and inflammatory markers upon consumption (Bested et al., 2013; Logan et al., 2003). Research has shown that gut microbes, in quantities undetectable by the immune system, can influence animal behaviour indicative of human stress (Logan and Katzman, 2005). This suggests that probiotics may have a beneficial influence on cognition and behaviour (Bested et al., 2013).

Conclusion

The evidence of the brain–gut bidirectional pathway is unequivocal, but the precise nature of the communication is still unknown. The way in which the gut affects psychopathology is still in its infancy, but evidence is starting to filter through. Impressive progress has been achieved in characterising the brain–gut axis, the clear majority of the research has been conducted using the animal model and progress in the human therapies has been much slower. Even though the bidirectional pathway linking the gut to the brain is well established, it still may be decades before mental healthcare professionals are able to give a single strain of probiotic bacteria which will prove clinically meaningful and long-lasting.

Throughout the preceding chapters theoretical positions will be advocated that build to draw a much clearer picture of the complexities of the symbiotic nature of the brain–gut interaction.

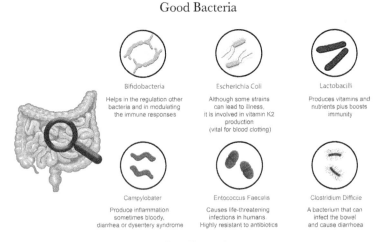

Figure 2   Good bacteria vs. Bad bacteria.

References

Ait-Belgnaoui A, Han W, Lamine F, Eutamene H, Fioramonti J, Bueno L and Theodorou V (2006) Lactobacillus farciminis treatment suppresses stress induced visceral hypersensitivity: a possible action through interaction with epithelial cell cytoskeleton contraction. Gut 55(8): 1090–1094. doi:10.1136/gut.2005.084194.

American Psychiatric Association (2000) Diagnostic and Statistical Manual of Mental Disorders, 4th Edition, Text Revised (DSM-IV-TR). Washington, DC: American Psychiatric Publishing.

American Psychiatric Association (2013) Diagnostic and Statistical Manual of Mental Disorders, 5th Edition. Washington, DC: American Psychiatric Publishing.

Bested AC, Logan AC and Selhub EM (2013) Intestinal microbiota, probiotics and mental health: from Metchnikoff to modern advances: Part I–autointoxication revisited. Gut Pathogens 5(1): 5. doi:10.1186/1757-4749-5-5.

Bezirtzoglou E (1997) The intestinal microflora during the first weeks of life. Anaerobe 3(2-3): 173–177. doi:10.1006/anae.1997.0102.

Colla J, Buka S, Harrington D and Murphy JM (2006) Depression and modernization. Social Psychiatry and Psychiatric Epidemiology 41(4): 271–279. doi:10.1007/s00127-006-0032-8.

Dinan TG and Quigley EM (2011) Probiotics in the treatment of depression: Science or science fiction? Australian and New Zealand Journal of Psychiatry 45(12): 1023–1025. doi:10.3109/00048674.2011.613766.

Emery R and Coan J (2010) What causes chest pain when feelings are hurt? Scientific American.

Fuller R (1989) Probiotics in man and animals. Journal of Applied Bacteriology 66(5): 365–378. doi:10.1111/j.1365-2672.1989.tb05105.x.

Fuller R (2012) Probiotics: the scientific basis. Springer Science & Business Media.

Furness JB and Costa M (1987) The enteric nervous system. Edinburgh: Churchill Livingstone.

Furness JB (2008) The enteric nervous system: normal functions and enteric neuropathies. Neurogastroenterology and Motility 20(s1): 32–38.

Gershon M (1998) The second brain: The scientific basis of gut instinct. New York: Harper Collins.

Hidaka BH (2012) Depression as a disease of modernity: explanations for increasing prevalence. Journal of Affective Disorders 140(3): 205–214. doi:10.1016/j.jad.2011.12.036.

Husebye E, Hellström PM, Sundler F, Chen J and Midtvedt T (2001) Influence of microbial species on small intestinal myoelectric activity and transit in germ-free rats. American Journal of Physiology-Gastrointestinal and Liver Physiology 280(3): G368–G380.

Logan A, Venket A and Irani D (2003) Chronic fatigue syndrome: lactic acid bacteria may be of therapeutic value. Medical Hypotheses 60(6): 915–923. doi:10.1016/S0306-9877(03)00096-3.

Logan A and Katzman M (2005) Major depressive disorder: probiotics may be an adjuvant therapy. Medical Hypotheses 64(3): 533–538. doi:10.1016/j.mehy.2004.08.019.

Logan A and Selhub E (2012) Vis Medicatrix naturae: does nature "minister to the mind"? Biopsychosocial Medicine 6(1): 11. doi:10.1186/1751-0759-6-11.

Mayer EA (2011) Gut feelings: the emerging biology of gut–brain communication. Nature Reviews Neuroscience 12(8): 453–466. doi:10.1038/nrn3071.

Mayer EA and Brunnhuber S (2012) Chapter 36—Gastrointestinal disorders. pp. 607–631. In: Michael FB, Aminoff J and Dick FS (Eds.). Handbook of Clinical Neurology (Vol. 106). Elsevier.

Mayer EA, Tillisch K and Gupta A (2015) Gut/brain axis and the microbiota. The Journal of Clinical Investigation 125(3): 926–938. doi:10.1172/JCI76304.

Mazmanian SK, Round JL and Kasper DL (2008) A microbial symbiosis factor prevents intestinal inflammatory disease. Nature 453(7195): 620–625. doi:10.1038/nature07008.

Metchnikoff E (1907) Lactic acid as inhibiting intestinal putrefaction. pp. 161–183. In: Heinemann W (Ed.). The Prolongation of Life: Optimistic Studies. London.

Parker R (1974) Probiotics, the other half of the antibiotic story. Animal Nutrition & Health 29(29): 4–8.

Pederson CS (1971) Microbiology of food fermentations. Microbiology of Food Fermentations.

Rhee S, Im E, Riegler M, Kokkotou E, O'Brien M and Pothoulakis C (2005) Pathophysiological role of Toll-like receptor 5 engagement by bacterial flagellin in colonic inflammation. Proceedings of the

National Academy of Sciences of the United States of America 102(38): 13610–13615. doi:10.1073/pnas.0502174102.

Rhee S, Pothoulakis C and Mayer E (2009) Principles and clinical implications of the brain–gut–enteric microbiota axis. Nature Reviews Gastroenterology and Hepatology 6(5): 306–314. doi:10.1038/nrgastro.2009.35.

Schlundt J (2001) Report of a Joint FAO/WHO Expert Consultation on Evaluation of Health and Nutritional Properties of Probiotics in Food Including Powder Milk with Live Lactic Acid Bacteria. Retrieved from https://web.archive.org/web/20121022161702/http://www.who.int/foodsafety/publications/fs_management/en/probiotics.pdf.

Tamime A (2002) Fermented milks: a historical food with modern applications—a review. European Journal of Clinical Nutrition 56(n4s): S2.

Tannock G, Munro K, Harmsen H, Welling G, Smart J and Gopal P (2000) Analysis of the fecal microflora of human subjects consuming a probiotic product containing Lactobacillus rhamnosus DR20. Applied and Environmental Microbiology 66(6): 2578–2588. doi:10.1128/AEM.66.6.2578-2588.

Turnbaugh PJ, Ley RE, Hamady M, Fraser-Liggett C, Knight R and Gordon JI (2007) The human microbiome project: exploring the microbial part of ourselves in a changing world. Nature 449(7164): 804. doi:10.1038/nature06244.

Vollaard E and Clasener H (1994) Colonization resistance. Antimicrobial Agents and Chemotherapy 38(3): 409.

CHAPTER 2

Probiotics and Chronic Fatigue Syndrome

Derek Larkin[1],* and *Colin R Martin*[2]

INTRODUCTION

Chronic fatigue syndrome (CFS) is the term that is generally accepted by clinicians to encompass the range of complaints that is also referred to as myalgic encephalomyelitis (ME) or chronic fatigue and immune dysfunction syndrome (Prins et al., 2006). CFS/ME is a complex condition with no known etiology, and is generally characterized by persistent and unexplained fatigue that cannot be relieved by rest and intensifies due to physical and mental activity (Christley et al., 2012). Patients presenting physical symptoms in which it is not possible to give a clear medical explanation is nothing new, such symptoms may include unexpected chest pains, dizziness, headaches, back pain, joint and muscle pains, bowel and bladder dysfunction, throat discomfort and chronic fatigue (London et al., 1997). CFS/ME is thought to affect about 0.3% of the population which amounts to about 972,000 individuals in the USA, and roughly 195,000 individuals in the UK. However, the prevalence is thought to be much higher because of the multifaceted ways in which the condition is diagnosed, as such the rate could be as high as 3.3% (Smith et al., 2015) therefore the actual figure could be as high as 10,692,000 individuals in the USA, and 2,145,000 individuals in the UK.

Given the multitude of symptoms that CFS/ME patients present with, treatment approaches have been broad including immunologic, pharmacologic, behavioral treatment and complementary and alternative medicines (Smith et al., 2015). No medications have been specifically developed for the treatment of CFS/ME, many treatments are off label (without specific review or approval) these generally treat the underlying symptoms such as pain, fatigue, autonomic dysfunction and sleep

[1] Edge Hill University, St Helens Road, Ormsirk, Lancashire, L39 4QP.
[2] Faculty of Society and Health, Buckinghamshire New University, Uxbridge Campus, 106 Oxford Road, Uxbridge, Middlesex, UB8 1NA, UK.
* Corresponding author

dysfunction. Some are treated with immune modulators, antiviral medication and antibiotics (FDA, 2013). In practice, the clinical management of patients varies widely and many patients receive a multifaceted approach to treatment (Smith et al., 2015).

The beneficial effects of probiotics are often disparate and strain specific (Ebel et al., 2014). Some species conferred beneficial effects for example, in the treatment of acute diarrhea associated with retrovirus (Isolauri et al., 1995), ulcerated colitis (Ishikawa et al., 2003) and Helicobacter pylori infection (Nista et al., 2004). Some studies report preventative effects, such as prevention of antibiotic associated diarrhea in children (Kunz et al., 2004). The commercial exploitation of probiotic products is still associated with a large body of unsubstantiated claims and many proposed health effects, and still needs additional investigation particularly in relation to the potential benefits for the health consumer, the main market for probiotic products. The perception that fermented milk yoghurt is beneficial is already widespread within many regions of the world, traditionally these products have been and are being used by local healers for treatment of such diverse conditions such as skin allergies, Stomach upsets, specifically diarrhea, and vaginal discharge (Senok et al., 2005). There is however major concern regarding quality, labelling and verification of claims to probiotic products. Studies have found in a number of probiotic products tested that they had incorrect labelling, markedly reduced numbers of probiotic strains, and worryingly the presence of strains not included on the labels including the potential pathogenic strain *Enterococcus faecium* (Senok et al., 2005). *Enterococcus faecium* has been associated with causing diseases such as neonatal meningitis or endocarditis. There has been a call for international consensus on evaluating the efficacy and safety of such products.

Several studies have started to explore the use of probiotics to help treat/alleviate some of the symptoms of CFS/ME (Sullivan et al., 2009). There is a growing

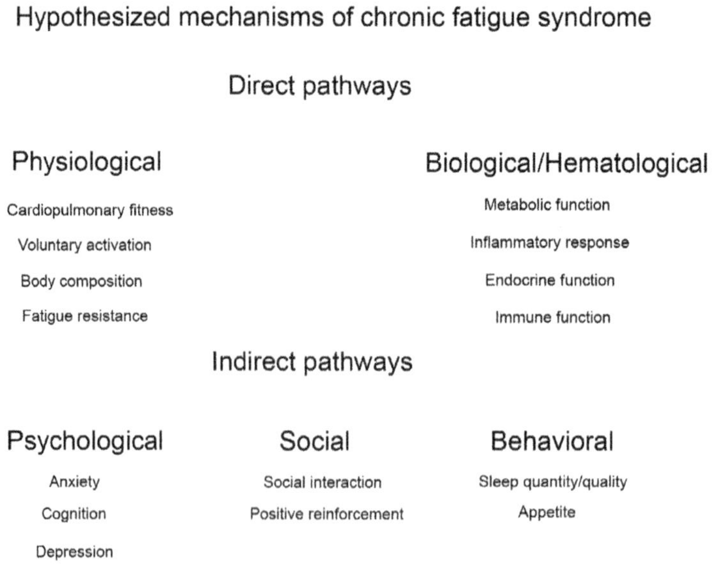

Hypothesized mechanisms of chronic fatigue syndrome

Direct pathways

Physiological	Biological/Hematological
Cardiopulmonary fitness	Metabolic function
Voluntary activation	Inflammatory response
Body composition	Endocrine function
Fatigue resistance	Immune function

Indirect pathways

Psychological	Social	Behavioral
Anxiety	Social interaction	Sleep quantity/quality
Cognition	Positive reinforcement	Appetite
Depression		

Figure 1 Hypothesized mechanisms of Chronic Fatigue Syndrome: (CRF). Adapted from McNeely and Courneya (2010).

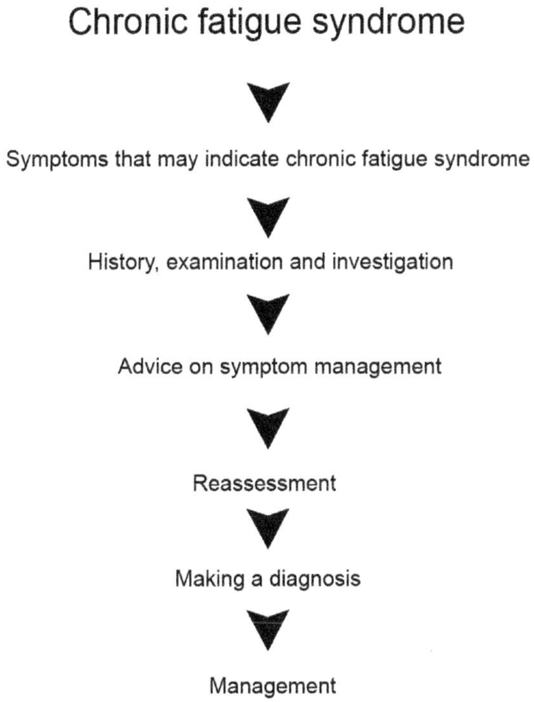

Chronic fatigue syndrome

Symptoms that may indicate chronic fatigue syndrome

History, examination and investigation

Advice on symptom management

Reassessment

Making a diagnosis

Management

Figure 2 Assessment and diagnosis of chronic fatigue syndrome NICE pathway: Adapted from National Institute for Health and Care Excellence 2016.

evidence base that suggests that CFS/ME is associated with discernable alterations in gut microbiota, with lower levels of *Bifidobacterium* and higher levels of aerobic bacteria (Logan et al., 2003).

Chronic Fatigue Syndrome/Myalgic Encephalomyelitis

Chronic fatigue syndrome (CFS)/myalgic encephalomyelitis (ME) is a debilitating multisystem condition characterized by chronic and disabling fatigue. Accompanied by several symptoms including pain, sleep disturbances, neurologic and cognitive changes, motor impairment and autoimmune and autonomic responses (Smith et al., 2015; Carruthers et al., 2003; Carruthers et al., 2011; Fukuda et al., 1994). There is a certain amount of uncertainty regarding the cause of CFS/ME, and whether it is a pathologically discrete syndrome (Carruthers et al., 2011), or whether ME should be considered a subset of CFS, or its own discrete disease (Jason et al., 2013) or whether symptoms are non-specific and shared by other disease entities (Smith et al., 2015).

Reports of CFS type patient cases were first described in the 19th and 20th centuries (Shorter, 2008) but it was not until the 1980's with the advent of ME that interest and research started to grow (Prins et al., 2006). In general terms, ME has two main symptoms, neurological and chronic fatigue. Because of the chronic fatigue symptomology comparisons were made with neurasthenia, and the possible role of viruses and microorganisms was examined (Bell and Mccartney, 1984; Prins et al.,

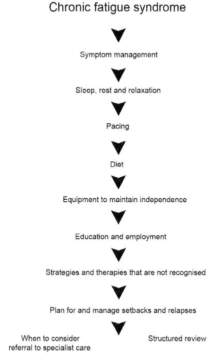

Figure 3 Management of chronic fatigue syndrome NICE pathway Adapted from National Institute for Health and Care Excellence 2016.

2006). In the absence of a medical explanation and recognizable physiological cause, ME has been described as a psychiatric disorder (Byrne, 1988), or the 20th century condition (Prins et al., 2006). Even now there is disagreement on a name chronic fatigue syndrome or myalgic encephalomyelitis, and diagnosis of CFS as an illness, and on the absence of underlying pathophysiology (Prins et al., 2006).

Early research exploring CFS were hampered by the lack of consistent diagnostic features and definitions. From 1988 several lines of research started to use case studies to develop definitions (Holmes et al., 1988; Sharpe et al., 1991; Lloyd et al., 1990). In an attempt to address the problem of case definition it was decided by Holmes et al. (1988) to settle on the name of chronic fatigue syndrome (CFS), because it was descriptive and free from unproven etiological implications (Sharpe et al., 1991). Holmes et al. (1988) also devised a definition of the syndrome, although welcomed at the time the definition proved to be unsatisfactory in practice (Manu et al., 1988). Difficulties arose from inadequate and poorly described sampling procedures, choice of comparison groups, shortcomings in study design and measures of poor or unspecified reliability (David et al., 1988). In 1991 Sharpe et al. organized a conference with the aim of seeking agreement amongst researchers on the conduct and report in the future studies of patients with chronic fatigue syndrome. This lead to more consistent methodologies, reporting of findings, and as a consequence the diagnosis of CFS is made on clinical criteria (Devanur and Kerr, 2006). The most widely accepted definition for the diagnosis of CFS was devised by the Centre for

Chronic fatigue syndrome

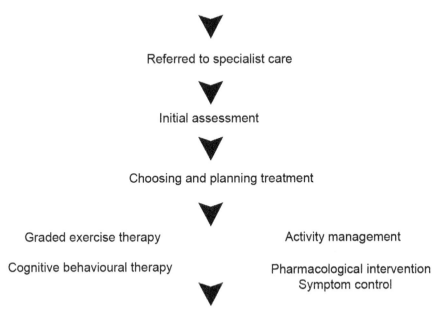

Referred to specialist care

Initial assessment

Choosing and planning treatment

Graded exercise therapy   Activity management

Cognitive behavioural therapy   Pharmacological intervention
                                                              Symptom control

Planning for and manage setbacks and relapses

Figure 4 Specialist care for chronic fatigue syndrome NICE pathway Adapted from National Institute for Health and Care Excellence 2016.

Disease Control (Fukuda et al., 1994). CFS is defined by several clinical features; clinically evaluated, unexplained persistent, or relapsing chronic fatigue of new or definite onset (not lifelong), not the result of ongoing exertion; not substantially alleviated by rest; resulting in substantial reduction in previous activities. There must also be concurrent presence of four or more of the following symptoms all of which must be persistent or recurred during the past 6 months of illness, and must not have pre-dated the fatigue; there must be self-reported impairment in short-term memory or concentration severe enough to cause substantial reduction in previous levels of occupation, education, social or personal activities; sore throat; tender cervical or axillary lymph nodes; muscle pain, multiple joint pain without joint swelling or redness; headaches of a new type, pattern or severity; unrefreshing sleep; post exertional malaise lasting longer than 24 hours (Devanur and Kerr, 2006). It is also vital to exclude physiological and psychiatric disease which may cause fatigue.

The hypothalamic-pituitary-adrenal (HPA) axis principal purpose is to maintain homoeostasis to physical and psychological stress. Disruption of HPA axis has been implicated in pathogenesis of CFS (Cleare, 2004). Studies have also found that cortisol (a steroid hormone in the glucocorticoid class of hormones, one action of cortisol is in the response to stress) is lower in patients with CFS (Poteliakhoff, 1981). It is suggested that initial stress may result in prolonged hyper-activation of the HPA axis which may lead to insensitivity or blunted response long-term (Devanur and Kerr, 2006). The relationship has been established between the immune system and the HPA axis. Interleukin 6 (IL-6, an interleukin that acts as both a pro-inflammatory cytokine and an anti-inflammatory myokine) has been shown to activate the HPA axis increasing plasma Adrenocorticotropic hormone (ATCH, also known as corticotrophin, and is known to be released in response to stress), and corticosteroid (steroid hormone, also known to be released in response to stress) in mice studies (Wang and Dunn, 1998). Interleukin 1 and 6 are known to synergistically active the HPA axis, thought to be activated during psychological stress (Zhou et al., 1993). Zhou et al. (1996) found the modulatory role for IL-6 stimulated HPA axis activity in response to IL-1 or a novelty psychological stressor, but not for restraint stress, which is known to cause anxiety and depression like behaviors, downregulates glucocorticoid receptor expression, and attenuates glutamate release induced by brain-derived neurotrophic factor in the prefrontal cortex (Chiba et al., 2012). It is therefore likely that HPA axis activation is not as a response of CFS, but is secondary to primary pathogenesis, at least in the initial stages of the condition (Devanur and Kerr, 2006). Even if there are no specific changes in the HPA axis as a direct action of CFS, the activation during the course of the condition might play a role in exacerbating or perpetuating symptoms late on in the course of the illness (Cleare, 2004). Emotional stress is known to play a significant role in the progression of CFS. Although multifaceted it is understood that emotional stress may result in various changes to the immune response to endogenous viral infections, emotional stress is also known to affect the HPA axis.

Gut Microbiota

The human gastrointestinal tract contains a complex, delicately balanced ecosystem of more than 17 bacterial family encompassing 400 to 500 different microbial species (Lakhan and Kirchgessner, 2010). *Lactobacillus, Bifidobacteria, Bacteroides, Clostridia, Fusobacteria, Eubacteria, Peptococcus, Streptococcus, Escherichia and Veillonella* are the main commensal bacteria. In general terms, these bacteria regulate a multitude of host processes, and provide essential nutrients. Under normal circumstances within healthy individuals with no underlying pathology, the guts microbial community is in equilibrium. However, these finely balanced bacterial communities can be altered by a number of factors (Jiménez, 2009). For example, clinical observations and animal experiments have suggested that intestinal bacteria trigger and perpetuate chronic bowel inflammation (Swidsinski et al., 2002). Individuals with Inflammatory bowel disease have increased bacteroides, adherence or invasive *Escherichia coli*, and enterococci, and reduced *Bifidobacteria* and *Lactobacillus* species (Swidsinski et al., 2002). Gut microbial community equilibrium can also be altered by psychological stress, which has been found to decrease the numbers of *Bifidobacteria* and *Lactobacillus*. Within an animal model psychological stress was applied to pregnant primates, and it was found that even moderate disturbances during pregnancy was sufficient to alter the intestinal microflora in the new-born infants, this was thought to leave the host with increased susceptibility to opportunistic infections (Bailey et al., 2004). Links are being made between stress, both psychological and physical exhaustion, and the onset of chronic fatigue syndrome (Maes et al., 2012).

Probiotics

Over the past few decades there has been a significant exploration on the characterization and verification of the potential health benefits associated with the use of probiotics (Senok et al., 2005). Probiotics are defined as live organisms that, when administered in adequate amounts conferred beneficial effects on the host (WHO, 2001). In recent years there's been an increase in research into probiotics as well as a growing commercial interest in probiotic food (Senok et al., 2005). The two main genera of gram positive bacteria, *Bifidobacteria* and *Lactobacillus,* are used extensively as probiotics (Holzapfel et al., 2001; WHO, 2001). However, other genera, such as *Escherichia*, *Enterococcus* and *Saccharomyces*, have also been marketed as probiotics (Holzapfel et al., 2001), although concerns still remain regarding the safe use of these organisms for this purpose (Ishibashi and Yamazaki, 2001).

Chronic Fatigue Syndrome and Probiotics

Alongside the chronic fatigue, CFS is characterized by numerous psychological disturbances for example, headaches, myalgia, arthralgia, and post-exertional malaise, cognitive difficulties, with poor memory or concentration; unrefreshing sleep and mood changes such as depression and anxiety (Wessely et al., 1998). In combination with these features patients will often complain of gastrointestinal disturbances, which may include abdominal pain or discomfort and alterations to bowel habit (Lakhan and Kirchgessner, 2010). Individuals are also likely to be given a previous diagnosis of irritable bowel syndrome, a common functional disorder of the gastrointestinal tract, and experience irritable bowel syndrome related symptoms (Aaron et al., 2000). Given the high frequency of comorbidities in CFS the underlying pathophysiological mechanisms cannot be confined to one particular organ (e.g., the brain or gut) but it has been argued the CFS must involve an integrated system or mechanism such as the brain–gut axis or the autonomic nervous system (Lakhan and Kirchgessner, 2010), although the precise pathophysiology of CFS is still unknown.

There is an increasing body of evidence describing the immune dysfunction in CFS, Fletcher et al. (2009) in which cytokines (small proteins, that are important in the immune response) abnormalities appear common. Cytokine abnormalities indicate immune activation and inflammation and point to potential therapeutic strategies. Studies appear to show a pro-inflammatory cytokine up regulation and down regulation of important mediators of cytotoxic cell function. However, the cytokine changes observed are likely to be more indicative of immune activation and inflammation, rather than specific to CFS. Nevertheless, cytokine abnormalities appear to be relatively common within individuals with chronic fatigue syndrome (Fletcher et al., 2009).

Probiotic lactic acid plays an essential role in food production and health maintenance; interest is increasing in this species of bacteria to discover potential health benefits associated with them (Quinto et al., 2014). Lactic acid bacteria are a group of Gram-positive (appear violet when stained) non-sporulating, anaerobic or facultative aerobic cocci or rods, which produces lactic acid as a main fermentation product of the metabolism of carbohydrates (Quinto et al., 2014). Four genera have been recognized as lactic acid bacteria *Lactobacillus, Leuconostoc, Pediococcus,* and *Streptococcus.*

There is emerging evidence which suggests that intestinal microflora in CFS is markedly different from in that of healthy individuals. Logan et al. (2003) advocate that this picture is not surprising given the overabundance of research citing the influence of stressors on microbial flora health, specifically *Lactobacilli, Bifidobacteria* and anaerobes. The loss in volume of these bacteria appears to amplify domination of TH2-type cytokines (influence anti-inflammatory immune response). This is important because TH1-type cytokines are a link in the production of a pro-inflammatory response; the optimal scenario would be an harmonious balance between TH1 and TH2, well suited to the immune challenge (Berger, 2000). Logan et al. (2003) argue that the administration of specific strains of lactic acid bacteria can help regulate the composition of intestinal flora and may have a significant impact on shifting the cytokine balance towards a TH1 driven cellular immunity. They also argue that lactic acid bacteria can protect the intestinal epithelial barrier and enhance the absorption of vitamins and minerals, particularly those that are deceased in CFS patients. It has also been argued that lactic acid bacteria may have the potential to act as a strong antioxidant in the patient population that is known to have increased oxidative stress and one that has diminished antioxidant capacity (Logan et al., 2003). Liz'ko (1987) has proposed that the administration of the *Bifidobacteria* can make dramatic alterations in the microflora of those under an emotional and physical stress, typically seen in patients with CFS. But stress comes in many forms, and it has been shown that regular exposure to excessive physical stress as well as nervous and emotional strain has the ability to change the composition of intestinal microflora, correction of microflora by means of *Bifidumbacterin*, a curative lactic fermentation alimentary product, appears to have the effect of restoring intestinal flora, and also has the ability of improving general state of the patients (Kafarskaia et al., 1992).

Lactic acid bacteria have been shown to decrease amine production; amines have been implicated in the neurotoxic effect associated with chronic fatigue syndrome (Modler et al., 1990). Many studies have found low levels of *Bifidobacteria* in patients with CFS, which is particularly important given that the available evidence suggests that specific groups of the lactic acid bacteria when changed or diminished indicate a state of unhealthiness (Logan et al., 2003). It would seem that microbes of the gastrointestinal tract are intricately involved in the systemic immune and nervous system, the part the systems play in the onset and maintenance of chronic fatigue syndrome is quite possibly underestimated.

Sullivan et al. (2009) report a study in which they investigated 15 individuals that fulfilled the criteria set by the international researchers in the field the US Centre for Disease Control and Prevention (see Fukuda et al., 1994). The patients had high disability and fatigue severity scores. During the first two weeks of the study baseline observations without treatment were assessed, after which four weeks of probiotic product was administered, followed by a four-week follow-up period. The aim of the study was to explore *Lactobacillus paracasei* ssp. *Paracasei* F19, *Lactobacillus acidophilus* NCFB 1748 and *Bifidobacterium lactis* Bb12 on fatigue and physical activity in CFS patients. *Lactobacillus paracasei* ssp. is a gram-positive species of lactic acid bacteria, and is used primarily in a dairy product fermentation process and in probiotic products. *Paracasei* F19 is also used in the fermentation of milk product and a probiotic. Sullivan found that even though there was no discernible change in gastrointestinal microflora, patients did report neurocognitive improvements. Seemingly indicating that the administration of probiotics may have a beneficial effect on some cognitive aspects of CFS, improving subjective reports of fatigue and mood after probiotic treatment.

In a report commissioned by the FDA (2013) patients with CFS were asked about their experience with symptoms, and the resulting impact symptoms exert on patients daily life. The psychological difficulties for individuals living with CFS are often thought secondary to the physiological symptoms. The effectiveness of probiotics supplementation to improve mental-health among populations with and without CFS is still within its infancy, however this area of research is starting to gather interest. Many of the patients acknowledge the emotional strain that CFS exerted on their daily activities. Many patients exhibit a broad range of symptoms, many reporting disturbances in their emotional realm, two of the most frequent reported non-physical symptoms was anxiety and depression (Rao et al., 2009). Observations reported within probiotic and CFS research have highlighted the importance of the interrelationship between gastrointestinal microbiota, the central nervous system and immune functioning in particular (Pirbaglou et al., 2016), but also the patients emotional state (FDA, 2013). Rao et al. (2009) found that the administration of *Lactobacillus casei* Shirota within a population of patients with CFS had two beneficial effects, one was to increase *Lactobacillus* and *Bifidobacteria* within the gut; secondly to significantly decrease the anxiety symptoms as measured on the Beck Depression Scale and also the Beck Anxiety Inventory. This study would suggest a possible mechanism whereby probiotics might influence anxiety and depression. These data would suggest that specific strain of probiotic bacteria may have a role in mediating some of the emotional symptoms of chronic fatigue syndrome and possibly other related conditions (Rao et al., 2009).

Conclusion

A prerequisite for therapeutic probiotic administration is based on the concept that the gut ecosystem contributes to human physiology, and the gut has an unequivocal connection to the brain and consequently its modulation by use of probiotics, may help maintain health and reduce the risk of disease. As we can see from the studies outlined above understanding the complexity of gut microbiota, and specific components associated with the progression of disease, particularly within chronic fatigue syndrome is rapidly increasing. However, the evidence on microbiome-mediated effects by intervention with classical probiotics on humans is however still extremely limited. It's clear from the evidence that treatments using probiotics for chronic fatigue syndrome principally moderate the symptoms of the condition but not the underlying pathology. There is however new and exciting research exploring new generations of probiotics, some of which may help the symptoms of chronic fatigue syndrome particularly around inflammation. These probiotics however need to be evaluated in clinical trials, but whether they would be effective on humans at a population level or in personalised programs of treatment remain to be explored.

Evidence supports the contention that intestinal dysbiosis or gastrointestinal dysfunction can profoundly affect multiple aspects of mood and cognitive function (Jackson et al., 2015). Both Rao et al. (2009) and Sullivan et al. (2009) found probiotic supplementation may have a beneficial effect on mood related symptoms associated with CFS, which is an argument much in line with Logan et al. (2003) who suggested that altered intestinal microbiota contributes to the pathogenesis of CFS, and that therapeutic rebalance or modification of intestinal microbiota may have the potential to reduce the symptoms. These studies appear to lend support to the notion that alterations in gut microbiota can change the subjective symptoms expressed by CFS patients. Studies also appear to show that the administration of specific strains of probiotic can ameliorate some of the symptoms of chronic fatigue syndrome.

Understanding the role of naturally occurring intestinal bacteria and the ecological interplay with human health and disease, has the potential to provide a robust rationale for selective probiotic strains intervention. These interventions may facilitate the optimisation of integrated dietary strategies to efficiency modulate the human gut microbiota towards beneficial nutrition in clinical, and home settings.

References

Aaron LA, Burke MM and Buchwald D (2000) Overlapping conditions among patients with chronic fatigue syndrome, fibromyalgia, and temporomandibular disorder. Archives of Internal Medicine 160: 221–227.

Bailey MT, Lubach GR and Coe CL (2004) Prenatal stress alters bacterial colonization of the gut in infant monkeys. Journal of Pediatric Gastroenterology and Nutrition 38: 414–421.

Bell EJ and Mccartney RA (1984) A study of coxsackie B virus infections, 1972–1983. Journal of Hygiene 93: 197–203.

Berger A (2000) Th1 and Th2 responses: what are they? BMJ 321: 424.

Byrne E (1988) Idiopathic chronic fatigue and myalgia syndrome (myalgic encephalomyelitis): some thoughts on nomenclature and aetiology. The Medical Journal of Australia 148: 80–82.

Carruthers BM, Jain AK, De Meirleir KL, Peterson DL, Kilmas NG, Lerner AM, Bested AC, Pierre Flor-Henry MB, Joshi P, Peter Powles AC, Sherkey JA and van de Sande MI (2003) Myalgic encephalomyelitis/chronic fatigue syndrome: clinical working case definition, diagnostic and treatment protocols. Journal of Chronic Fatigue Syndrome 11: 7–115.

Carruthers BM, van de Sande MI, De Meirleir KL, Kilmas NG, Broderick G, Mitchell T, Staines D, Powles ACP, Speight N, Vallings R, Bateman L, Baumgarten-Austrheim B, Bell DS, Carlo-Stella N, Chia J, Darragh A, Jo D, Lewis D, Light AR, Marshall-Gradisbik S, Mena I, Mikovits JA, Miwa K, Murovska M, Pall ML and Stevens S (2011) Myalgic encephalomyelitis: international consensus criteria. Journal of Internal Medicine 270: 327–338.

Chiba S, Numakawa T, Ninomiya M, Richards MC, Wakabayashi C and Kungi H (2012) Chronic restraint stress causes anxiety- and depression-like behaviors, downregulates glucocorticoid receptor expression, and attenuates glutamate release induced by brain-derived neurotrophic factor in the prefrontal cortex. Progress in Neuro-Psychopharmacology and Biological Psychiatry 39: 112–119.

Christley Y, Martin CJH and Martin CR (2012) Perinatal perspectives on chronic fatigue syndrome. British Journal of Midwifery 20: 389–393.

Cleare AJ (2004) The HPA axis and the genesis of chronic fatigue syndrome. Trends in Endocrinology and Metabolism 15: 55–59.

David AS, Wessely S and Pelosi AJ (1988) Postviral fatigue syndrome: time for a new approach. British Medical Journal (Clinical Research Ed.) 296: 696–699.

Devanur LD and Kerr JR (2006) Chronic fatigue syndrome. Journal of Clinical Virology 37: 139–150.

Ebel B, Lemetais G, Beney L, Cachon R, Sokol H, Langella P and Gervais P (2014) Impact of probiotics on risk factors for cardiovascular diseases. A review. Critical Reviews in Food Science and Nutrition 54: 175–189.

FDA (2013) The Voice of the Patient. A series of reports from the U.S. Food and Drug Administration's (FDA's) Patient-Focused Drug Development Initiative. Available at: http://www.fda.gov/downloads/ForIndustry/UserFees/PrescriptionDrugUserFee/UCM368806.pdf.

Fletcher MA, Zeng XR, Barnes Z, Levis S and Kilmas NG (2009) Plasma cytokines in women with chronic fatigue syndrome. Journal of Translational Medicine 7: 1.

Fukuda K, Straus SE, Hickie I, Sharpe MC, Dobbins JG, Komaroff A (1994) The chronic fatigue syndrome: a comprehensive approach to its definition and study. Annals of Internal Medicine 121: 953–959.

Holmes GP, Kaplan JE, Gantz NM, Komraff AL, Schonberger LB, Straus SE, Jones JF, Dubois RE, Cunningham-Rundles C and Pawha S (1988) Chronic fatigue syndrome: a working case definition. Annals of Internal Medicine 108: 387–389.

Holzapfel WH, Haberer P, Geisen R, Bjokroth J and Schillinger U (2001) Taxonomy and important features of probiotic microorganisms in food and nutrition. The American Journal of Clinical Nutrition 73: 365s–373s.

Ishibashi N and Yamazaki S (2001) Probiotics and safety. The American Journal of Clinical Nutrition 73: 465s–470s.

Ishikawa H, Akedo I, Umesaki Y, Tanaka R, Imaoka A and Otani T (2003) Randomized controlled trial of the effect of bifidobacteria-fermented milk on ulcerative colitis. Journal of the American College of Nutrition 22: 56–63.

Isolauri E, Joensuu J, Suomalainen H, Luomala M and Veslkari T (1995) Improved immunogenicity of oral D x RRV reassortant rotavirus vaccine by *Lactobacillus casei* GG. Vaccine 13: 310–312.

Jackson ML, Butt H, Ball M, Lewis DP and Bruck D (2015) Sleep quality and the treatment of intestinal microbiota imbalance in Chronic Fatigue Syndrome: A pilot study. Sleep Science 8: 124–133.

Jason LA, Brown A, Evans M, Sunnquist M and Newton JL (2013) Contrasting chronic fatigue syndrome versus myalgic encephalomyelitis/chronic fatigue syndrome. Fatigue: Biomedicine, Health & Behavior 1: 168–183.

Jiménez MB (2009) Treatment of irritable bowel syndrome with probiotics. An etiopathogenic approach at last. Rev Esp Enferm Dig (Madrid) 101: 553–564.

Kafarskaia L, Glad'ko I, Efimov B, Tarabrina NP, Skvorlsov VM and Korshunov VM (1992) The effect of fermented-milk bifidumbacterin on the intestinal microflora of test pilots. Zhurnal mikrobiologii, epidemiologii, i immunobiologii: 12–14.

Kunz AN, Noel JM and Fairchok MP (2004) Two cases of Lactobacillus bacteremia during probiotic treatment of short gut syndrome. Journal of Pediatric Gastroenterology and Nutrition 38: 457–458.

Lakhan SE and Kirchgessner A (2010) Gut inflammation in chronic fatigue syndrome. Nutrition & Metabolism 7: 1–10.

Liz'ko N (1987) The dysbacteriosis of extreme states. Antibiotiki i meditsinskaia biotekhnologiia= Antibiotics and medical biotechnology/Ministerstvo meditsinskoi promyshlennosti SSSR 32: 184–186.

Lloyd AR, Hickie I, Boughton CR, Spencer O and Wakefield D (1990) Prevalence of chronic fatigue syndrome in an Australian population. The Medical Journal of Australia 153: 522–528.

Logan AC, Venket Rao A and Irani D (2003) Chronic fatigue syndrome: lactic acid bacteria may be of therapeutic value. Medical Hypotheses 60: 915–923.

London RCoPo, Psychiatrists RCo and Practitioners RCoG (1997) Chronic Fatigue Syndrome: report of a joint working group of the Royal Colleges of Physicians, Psychiatrists and General Practitioners. Royal College of Physicians.

Maes M, Twisk FNM, Kubera M, Ringel K, Lewis JC and Geffard M (2012) Increased IgA responses to the LPS of commensal bacteria is associated with inflammation and activation of cell-mediated immunity in chronic fatigue syndrome. J Affect Disord 136: 909–917.

Manu P, Lane TJ and Matthews DA (1988) The frequency of the chronic fatigue syndrome in patients with symptoms of persistent fatigue. Annals of Internal Medicine 109: 554–556.

McNeely ML and Courneya KS (2010) Exercise programs for cancer-related fatigue: evidence and clinical guidelines. Journal of the National Comprehensive Cancer Network 8(8): 945–953.

Modler H, McKellar R and Yaguchi M (1990) Bifidobacteria and bifidogenic factors. Canadian Institute of Food Science Technology Journal 23: 29–41.

Nista EC, Candelli M, Cremonini F, Cazzato IA, Zocco MA, Franceschi F, Cammarota G, Gasbarrini G and Gasbarrini A (2004) Bacillus clausii therapy to reduce side-effects of anti-Helicobacter pylori treatment: randomized, double-blind, placebo controlled trial. Alimentary Pharmacology and Therapeutics 20: 1181–1188.

Pirbaglou M, Katz J, de Souza RJ, Stearns JC, Motamed M and Rivto P (2016) Probiotic supplementation can positively affect anxiety and depressive symptoms: a systematic review of randomized controlled trials. Nutrition Research 36: 889–898.

Poteliakhoff A (1981) Adrenocortical activity and some clinical findings in acute and chronic fatigue. Journal of Psychosomatic Research 25: 91–95.

Prins JB, van der Meer JWM and Bleijenberg G (2006) Chronic fatigue syndrome. The Lancet 367: 346–355.

Quinto EJ, Jiménez P, Caro I, Tejero J, Mateo J and Gribes T (2014) Probiotic lactic acid bacteria: A review. Food and Nutrition Sciences 5: 1765.

Rao AV, Bested AC, Beaulne TM, Katzman MA, Lorio C, Beradi JM and Logano AC (2009) A randomized, double-blind, placebo-controlled pilot study of a probiotic in emotional symptoms of chronic fatigue syndrome. Gut Pathogens 1: 6.

Senok A, Ismaeel A and Botta G (2005) Probiotics: facts and myths. Clinical Microbiology and Infection 11: 958–966.

Sharpe M, Archard L, Banatvala J, Borysiewicz LK, Clare AW, David A, Edwards RH, Hawton KE, Lambert HP and Lane RJ (1991) A report—chronic fatigue syndrome: guidelines for research. Journal of the Royal Society of Medicine 84: 118.

Shorter E (2008) From paralysis to fatigue: a history of psychosomatic illness in the modern era. Simon and Schuster.

Smith MB, Haney E, McDonagh M, Pappas M, Daeges M, Wasson N, Fu R and Nelson HD (2015) Treatment of myalgic encephalomyelitis/chronic fatigue syndrome: a systematic review for a National Institutes of Health Pathways to Prevention Workshop. Annals of Internal Medicine 162: 841–850.

Sullivan Å, Nord CE and Evengård B (2009) Effect of supplement with lactic-acid producing bacteria on fatigue and physical activity in patients with chronic fatigue syndrome. Nutrition Journal 8: 4.

Swidsinski A, Ladhoff A, Pernthaler A, Swidsinski S, Loeing-Baucke V, Ortner M, Weber J, Hoffman J, Schreiber S, Dietel M and Lochs H (2002) Mucosal flora in inflammatory bowel disease. Gastroenterology 122: 44–54.

Wang J and Dunn AJ (1998) Mouse interleukin-6 stimulates the HPA axis and increases brain tryptophan and serotonin metabolism. Neurochemistry International 33: 143–154.

Wessely S, Sharpe M and Hotopf M (1998) Chronic fatigue and its syndromes. Oxford University Press.

WHO F (2001) Evaluation of health and nutritional properties of powder milk and live lactic acid bacteria. Food and Agriculture Organization of the United Nations and World Health Organization Expert Consultation Report 1–34.

Zhou D, Kusnecov AW, Shurin MR, DePaoli M and Rabin BS (1993) Exposure to physical and psychological stressors elevates plasma interleukin 6: relationship to the activation of hypothalamic-pituitary-adrenal axis. Endocrinology 133: 2523–2530.

Zhou D, Shanks N, Riechman S, Liang R, Kusnecov AW and Rabin BS (1996) Interleukin 6 modulates interleukin-1- and stress-induced activation of the hypothalamic-pituitary-adrenal axis in male rats. Neuroendocrinology 63: 227–236.

Chapter 3

The Gut Microbiota, Health and Exercise

Marie Clare Grant[1,]* and *Julien S Baker*[2]

INTRODUCTION

Non-communicable disease and mental health disorders pose a substantial threat to global health. It is estimated that 450 million people worldwide are affected by a mental health disorder thus substantially contributing to the global health burden (WHO, 2017). In the UK, just under 20% of the population over 16 years have shown symptoms of anxiety or depression (female = 22.5%; male = 16.8%) (Mental Health Foundation, 2016). Globally, 63% of all deaths in 2008 were due to non-communicable disease, primarily cardiovascular disease, diabetes, cancer and chronic respiratory disease (Alwan et al., 2010). In the UK, nearly 3.6 million people have been diagnosed with diabetes (with another 1 million estimated to have undiagnosed type II diabetes) (Diabetes UK, 2016). Over the last decade the prevalence of cardiovascular disease has declined, however, in 2014 it was still the second biggest cause of death, after cancer, accounting for 27% of all deaths (British Heart Foundation, 2015).

Within contemporary society there are high levels of co-morbidity between mental health disorders and chronic medical conditions (Forsythe et al., 2010). For example, depression is strongly associated with obesity, hypertension, dyslipidaemia, metabolic syndrome and diabetes (Chengappa et al., 2004; Heiskanen et al., 2006). All the afore mentioned conditions are also linked to physical inactivity (Stohle, 2009). With such high prevalence of both mental health disorders and non-communicable

[1] Abertay University.
[2] University of the West of Scotland.
* Corresponding author: marieclare.grant@abertay.ac.uk

physical disease any potential adjunctive therapy to traditional medication must be considered. There is reasonable evidence to suggest the use probiotics and/or exercise can improve mental health conditions through alteration of the gut microbiota (Logan et al., 2005; Poole et al., 2011) and that exercise can play a vital role in the prevention of various non-communicable disease (Strohle, 2009).

The Gut Microbiota

The human gut microbiota is unique to each individual (Cerda et al., 2016) and comprised of trillions of microbes including bacteria, viruses and fungi. (Cronin et al., 2017). Within the gastro-intestinal (GI) tract of an adult human there are at least 160 prevalent bacterial species from a pool of 1000–1150 (Desbonnet et al., 2009). By the age of 12 months each individual develops a unique bacterial profile (Forsythe et al., 2010), however, through endogenous and exogenous influences, such as genetics, diet, lifestyle and antibiotics, the composition of the microbiota evolves and changes throughout life (Cerda et al., 2016).

Within an adult microbiota, in the Bacteria domain, 60–80 % of the phylotypes belong to *Firmicute* phyla and 15–30% to the *Bacteroidete* phyla (Ley et al., 2006). Other bacteria present belong to *Proteobacteria, Actinobacteria, Fusobacteria,* and *Verrucomicrobia* phyla (Robles et al., 2013). Non-communicable diseases, including obesity and metabolic syndrome, are associated with an altered gut microbiota (Cronin et al., 2017; Monda et al., 2017) with changes in the ratio between *Firmicutes* (increase) and *Bacteroidetes* (decrease) being specifically linked to obesity (Cerda et al., 2016).

The gut microbiota is also essential in the development of the immune system and can have a role in reducing the risk of developing diseases such as colon cancer and type II diabetes. Certain species of bacteria in the gut can also have an important role in various other mechanisms including the absorption of vitamins and minerals, lowering cholesterol, improving lactose tolerance and fermenting indigestible fibre (Quigley, 2013).

Probiotic Bacteria

Probiotic bacteria are known as the friendly bacteria within GI tract (Gleeson, 2006). They exist alongside neutral and pathogenic bacteria (Messaoudi et al., 2001).

> *Probiotic—'Supporting or Favouring Life'*
> (Lilly and Stillwell, 1965)

It has been known for several years that probiotic bacteria can positively impact the health of the individual (Bravo et al., 2012) with the first record being in 76BC by a Roman historian who acknowledged that fermented milk could be used to treat GI disturbances (Bottazzi, 1983). To be classed as a probiotic, bacteria must meet a number of essential criteria which are outlined as viability during processing, transport and storage; the ability to survive gastric transport; the ability to adhere to and colonise the GI tract; the ability to antagonise pathogenic bacteria and the demonstration of clinical health outcomes (West et al., 2009).

With relatively few commonly consumed food sources naturally containing probiotics, in contemporary society probiotics are added to many cultured dairy products (Ohashi and Ushida, 2007). Due to the recognised health benefits the most common strains of probiotic bacteria to be added to products for human consumptions belong to the species *Lactobacillus* sp. (of the *Firmicute* phyla) and *Bifidobacterium* sp. (of the *Actinobacteria* phyla) (Benton et al., 2007). In particular, as outlined by Cerda and colleagues (2016), *Lactobacillus* sp. and *Bifidobacterium* sp. in the gut have been found to enhance the absorption of vitamins (such as B and K) and minerals, improve lactate tolerance, have anti-diabetic effects, lower cholesterol, increase resistance to infection, decrease the risk of colon cancer (Kumar et al., 2012; Zhu et al., 2011), exert anti-inflammatory effects (Villena and Kitazawa, 2014) and produce short chain fatty acids (Logan et al., 2003).

Probiotics and Mood State

It is widely recognised that probiotics can positively influence mood state (Forsythe et al., 2010) due to the effect they can have on both anatomical connections such as the vagus nerve and humoral components such as the immune system and hypothalamus-pituitary-adrenal (HPA) axis (Bravo et al., 2012).

The vagus nerve is essential for communication between the bacteria, the gut and the brain (Desbonnet et al., 2009). This microbiota-gut-brain axis allows for bidirectional communication whereby the gut can influence changes in the brain and vice versa (Mayer et al., 2006) with any dysfunction in the axis linked to alterations in pain perception, emotion and overall wellbeing (Rhee et al., 2009). In terms of humoral response, activation of the HPA axis causes corticotrophin-releasing factor (CRF) to be released from the hypothalamus, adrenocorticotrophic hormone (ACTH) to be released from the pituitary and cortisol to be released from the adrenal glands (Cryan and Dinan, 2012). When cortisol is chronically elevated it can have a negative impact on factors such as immune function, glucose metabolism and mood. Therefore, impairment of the HPA system is linked to both stress and depression (Belmaker and Agam, 2008).

The beneficial effects of probiotics has been shown in rodents whose vagus nerve was cut. A strain of probiotic, *L. rhamnosus* (JB.1), was found to reduce stress induced elevation in corticosterone, however these effects were not evident in the vagotomised mice (Bravo et al., 2011).

In terms of human studies investigating the link between the gut microbiota and mood disorders most evidence suggests that there is significant improvement in mood disorders with the consumption of probiotics. For example, Rao et al. (2009) investigated the effect of a lactic acid probiotic on patients with chronic fatigue syndrome and associated depression and anxiety. Following the consumption of a probiotic containing a strain of *Lactobacillus* three times per day for eight weeks the treatment group were found to have a significant improvement in anxiety scores. More recently the effects of a multispecies probiotic on cognitive reactivity to sad mood were investigated. It was found that those who consumed the probiotic over a four week period significantly reduced their cognitive reactivity to sad mood, which is important due to the risk of sad mood developing into clinical depression (Steenbergen et al., 2015). It has been suggested that the effects of probiotics on anxiety and depression may be due to the competitive exclusion of detrimental gut pathogens, decreases in pro-inflammatory cytokines and communication with the central nervous system via vagal sensory fibres leading to changes in neurotransmitter levels or function (Messaaoudi et al., 2011).

Gut Microbiota, Obesity and Physical Activity

Obesity

The link between the gut microbiota and body fat has been demonstrated both in animal and human studies. Germ-free mice were found to have 40% less body fat than normal mice despite an increased food consumption. When the microbiota of the normal mice was transplanted into the germ free mice there was increase in body fat by 60% over a two week period. The authors suggested that the microbiota promotes monosaccharide absorption resulting in *de novo* hepatic lipogenesis (conversion of surplus energy to fat) and concluded that the gut microbiota is an important environmental factor which can affect energy storage of the host organism (Backhed et al., 2004).

The role of gut microbiota in the development of obesity has also been shown in humans. Through analysis of faecal microbiota, it has been found that obese humans have higher levels of *Firmicutes* and lower levels of *Bacteroides* when compared to samples taken from lean individuals. This ratio has, however, been found to be reversible though the implementation of a calorie controlled diet (Ley et al., 2006). These obesity related changes in the gut microbiota can influence several metabolic functions including lipid and carbohydrate metabolism and hepatic triglyceride production (Backhed et al., 2004; Quigley, 2013).

Therefore, there is compelling evidence to suggest that the gut microbiota can influence metabolism and so energy storage. This is important due to obesity leading to the development of various non-communicable conditions and mental health conditions.

Exercise

It is known that exercise has a crucial role in maintaining a healthy lifestyle and reducing the risk of developing various non-communicable medical conditions and/ or mood disorders (Strohle, 2009). However, a potential benefit of exercise which has been somewhat overlooked is the role it may play in developing a healthy gut microbiota. It has been proposed that physical activity through childhood and adolescence can result in a diverse microbiota which is linked good psychological and metabolic health (Mika and Fleshner, 2016). It may also be that uptake of regular physical activity in adulthood, leading to an improvement in cardiorespiratory fitness, can also have positive role in the alteration of the gut microbiota (Bermon et al., 2015; Cronin et al., 2017; Mika et al., 2015).

It has been suggested that the relationship between exercise and the gut microbiota may be bi-directional whereby the microbiota may be altered by exercise and exercise performance may be affected by the microbiota due to the effects it has on food digestion and absorption (Marroquin and Willoughby, 2017). The exact mechanisms whereby exercise may influence the microbiota are not fully understood, however, it has been proposed that exercise may influence several factors which in turn cause changes in the microbiota. Among these possible mechanisms include alteration in the bile acid profile, changes in the short-chain fatty acid profile, an increase in cytokine production and decrease in gut transit time (Cerda et al., 2016).

Despite the recent increase in research into the effects of exercise on the gut microbiota, as outlined by Cronin et al. (2017) there are two factors which make it difficult to establish the true relationship between the two variables. These are, (1) The influence of dietary changes (intentional or subconscious) which can often occur with changes in physical activity. (2) The unknown effects that dietary supplements such as energy bars, caffeine and protein have on the gut microbiota.

Results from animal studies suggest that exercise does promote positive changes in the microbiota. For example, Queipo-Ortuño et al. (2013) found that exercised rats had increased levels of *Lactobacillus* and *Blautia coccoides–Eubacterium*. It is only in the last few years that the role of exercise in the modification of the gut microbiota has been investigated in humans. One of the first studies to investigate the modification of the gut microbiota via exercise was conducted by Clarke et al. (2014) who found that within the gut microbiota of elite rugby players there was greater diversity of microbial species, particularly in the *Firmicute* phyla. This was positively correlated with protein intake and creatine kinase levels. Cardiorespiratory fitness has also been found to be positively correlated with a diverse gut microbiota with fitter individuals having increased butyrate production (an indicator of good gut health) (Estaki et al., 2016)

Recently Ibrahim and colleagues conducted two studies linked to exercise, probiotics and the gut microbiota. In the first of these studies the effect of probiotic supplementation and circuit training on immune response in sedentary young males was investigated (Ibrahim et al., 2017a). The main findings to emerge from this study was that 12 weeks of circuit training (3 times per week) improved immune cell count. However, there were no positive effects linked to probiotic supplementation (2 times per week for 12 weeks). Within the second study, the effects of circuit training and probiotics on muscular strength and power and cytokine response was investigated. Using a similar 12 week intervention, it was found that circuit training and circuit training combined with probiotic supplementation improved muscular strength and power. It was also found that interleukin (IL)-10 concentration significantly increased in the probiotics only group and the circuit training only group, with a non-significant increase in the group which combined circuit training with probiotic supplementation (Ibrahim et al., 2017b).

Finally, Allen et al. (2017) investigated the effect of 6 weeks of endurance exercise on the gut microbiota in previously sedentary lean and obese humans. Despite the two groups having different gut microbiota compositions prior to the exercise intervention, it was that without any changes in diet, the six week exercise period altered the gut microbiota and microbial-derived SCFAs in both lean and obese individuals. The changes however were strongly associated with body composition changes in lean participants and an increased VO_{2max} in obese participants.

Conclusion

On the basis of current evidence it can be suggested that the gut microbiota can be positively altered in humans through physical activity. This provides further evidence for physical activity to be prescribed as an adjunctive therapy for both mental health disorder and non-communicable disease. It also seems reasonable to advocate the use of probiotic supplementation to enhance the profile of the gut microbiota.

For Further Information in this area Please refer to:

Grant, MC and Baker, JS (2017) An overview of the effect of probiotics and exercise on mood and associated health conditions. Critical Reviews in Food Science and Nutrition 57(18): 3887–3893.

References

Allen JM, Mailing LJ, Niemiro GM, Moore R, Cook MD, White BA, Holscher HD and Woods JA (2017) Exercise Alters Gut Microbiota Composition and Function in Lean and Obese Humans. Medicine and Science in Sports and Exercise. doi: 10.1249/MSS.0000000000001495.

Alwan A, MacLean DR, Riley LM, Tursan d'Espaignet E, Mathers CD, Stevens GA and Bettcher D (2010) Monitoring and surveillance of chronic noncommunicable diseases: progress and capacity in high-burden countries. The Lancet 376: 1861–1868.

Backhed F, Ding H, Wang T, Hooper LV, Koh GY, Nagy A, Semenkovich CF and Gordon JI (2004) The gut microbiota as an environmental factor that regulates fat storage. Proceeding of the National Academy of Science USA 101: 15718–15723.

Belmaker RH and Agam G (2008) Major depressive disorder. New England Journal of Medicine 358: 55–68.

Benton D, Williams C and Brown A (2007) Impact of consuming a milk drink containing a probiotic on mood and cognition. European Journal of Clinical Nutrition 61: 355–361.

Bermon S, Petriz B, Kajeniene A, Prestes J, Castell L and Franco OL (2015) The microbiota: an exercise immunology perspective Exercise Immunology Review 21: 70–79.

Bravo JA, Forsythe P, Chew MV, Escaravage E, Savignac HM, Dinan TG, Bienenstock J and Cryan JF (2011) Ingestion of Lactobacillus strain regulates emotional behavior and central GABA receptor expression in a mouse via the vagus nerve. Proceedings of the National Academy of Sciences 108(38): 16050–16055.

Bravo JA, Julio-Pieper M, Forsythe P, Kunze W, Dinan TG, Bienenstock J and Cryan JF (2012) Communication between gastrointestinal bacteria and the nervous system. Current Option in Pharmacology 12: 1–6.

Bottazzi V (1983) Other fermented dairy products. Biotechnology. Weinhein: Verlag Chemie pp. 315–363.

British Heart Foundation (2015) Cardiovascular Disease. Available from: https://www.bhf.org.uk/research/heart-statistics [Accessed 12 December 2017].

Cerdá B, Pérez M, Pérez-Santiago JD, Tornero-Aguilera JF, González-Soltero R and Larrosa M (2016) Gut microbiota modification: another piece in the puzzle of the benefits of physical exercise in health? Frontiers in Physiology 7: 51. doi: 10.3389/fphys.2016.00051.

Chengappa K, Kupfer D, Parepally H, John V, Basu R, Buttenfield J, Schlict P, Houck P, Brar J and Gershon S (2004) The prevalence of the metabolic syndrome in patients with schizoaffective disorder-bipolar subtype. Bipolar Disorders 6: 314–318.

Clarke SF, Murphy EF, O'Sullivan O, Lucey AJ, Humphreys M, Hogan A et al. (2014) Exercise and associated dietary extremes impact on gut microbial diversity. Gut 63: 1913–1920. doi: 10.1136/gutjnl-2013-306541.

Cronin O, O'sullivan O, Barton W, Cotter PD, Molloy MG and Shanahan F (2017) Gut microbiota: implications for sports and exercise medicine. British Journal of Sports Medicine doi.org/10.1136/bjsports-2016-097225.

Cryan JF and Dinan TG (2012) Mind-altering microorganisms: the impact of the gut microbiota on brain and behaviour. Nature Reviews Neuroscience 13(10): 710–712.

Desbonnet L, Garrett L, Clarke G, Bienestock J and Dinan T (2009) The probiotic Bifidobacteria infantis: An assessment of potential antidepressant properties in the rat. Journal of Psychiatric Research 43: 164–174.

Diabetes UK (2016) Diabetes Prevalence 2016. Available from: https://www.diabetes.org.uk/professionals/position-statements-reports/statistics/diabetes-prevalence-2016 [Accessed 12 December 2017].

Estaki M, Pither J, Baumeister P, Little JP, Gill SK, Ghosh S, et al. (2016) Cardiorespiratory fitness as a predictor of intestinal microbial diversity and distinct metagenomic functions. Microbiome 4(1): 42. doi: 10.1186/s40168-016-0189-7.

Forsythe P, Sudo N, Dinan T, Taylor VH and Bienenstock J (2010) Mood and gut feelings. Brain, Behaviour and Immunity 24: 9–16.

Gleeson M (2006) Exercise, nutrition and immune function II. Micronutrients, antioxidants and other supplements. pp. 183–203. *In*: Gleeson M (Ed.). Immune Function in Sport and Exercise. Elsevier, China.

Heiskanen TH, Niskanen LK, Hintikka JJ, Koivumaa-Honkanen HT, Honkalampi KM, Haatainen KM and Viinamäki HT (2006) Metabolic syndrome and depression: a cross-sectional analysis. The Journal of Clinical Psychiatry 67(9): 1422–1427.

Ibrahim NS, Ooi FK, Chen CK and Muhamad AS (2017a) Effects of probiotics supplementation and circuit training on immune responses among sedentary young males. The Journal of Sports Medicine and Physical Fitness. doi: 10.23736/S0022-4707.17.07742-8.

Ibrahim NS, Muhamad AS, Ooi FK, Meor-Osman J and Chen CK (2017b) The effects of combined probiotic ingestion and circuit training on muscular strength and power and cytokine responses in young males. Applied Physiology, Nutrition, and Metabolism. doi: 10.1139/apnm-2017-0464.

Kumar RS, Kanmani P, Yuvaraj N, Paari KA, Pattukumar V, Thirunavukkarasu C et al. (2012) Lactobacillus plantarum AS1 isolated from south Indian fermented food Kallappam suppress 1,2-dimethyl hydrazine (DMH)-induced colorectal cancer in male Wistar rats. Applied Biochemistry and Biotechnology 166: 620–631.

Ley RE, Turnbaugh PJ, Klein S and Gordon JI (2006) Microbial ecology: human gut microbes associated with obesity. Nature 444: 1022–1023.

Lilly DM and Stillwell RH (1965) Probiotics: Growth promoting factors produced by micro-organisms. Science 147: 747–748.

Logan A, Rao V and Irani D (2003) Chronic fatigue syndrome: lactic acid bacteria may be of therapeutic value. Med Hypotheses 60: 915–923.

Logan AC and Katzman M (2005) Major depressive disorder: probiotics may be an adjuvant therapy. Medical Hypotheses 64: 533–538.

Marroquin F and Willoughby D (2017) Exercise and dietary factors affecting the microbiota: current knowledge and future perspectives. Journal of Nutritional Health and Food Engineering. 6(3): 00199 doi: 10.15406/jnhfe.207.06.00199.

Mayer EA, Tillisch K and Bradesi S (2006) Review article: modulation of the brain–gut axis as a therapeutic approach in gastrointestinal disease. Alimentary Pharmacology and Therapeutics 24: 919–933.

Mental Health Foundation (2016) Mental Health Statistics: UK and Worldwide. Available from: https://www.mentalhealth.org.uk/statistics/mental-health-statistics-uk-and-worldwide [Accessed 14 December 2017].

Messaoudi M, Lalonde R, Violle N, Herve J, Desor D, Nejdi A, Bisson JH, Rouget C, Pichelin M, Cazaubiel M and Cazaubiel JM (2011) Assessment of psychotropic-like properties of a probioticformulation (Lactobacillus helveticus R0052 and Bifidobacterium longum R0175) in rats and human subjects. British Journal of Nutrition 105: 755–764.

Mika A, Van Treuren W, Gonzalez A, Herrera J, Knight R, Fleshner (2015) Exercise is more effective at altering gut microbial composition and producing stable changes in lean mass in juvenile versus adult male F344 rats. PLoS One 10(5): e0125889.

Mika A and Fleshner M (2016) Early-life exercise may promote lasting brain and metabolic health through gut bacterial metabolites. Immunology and Cell Biology 94: 151–7.

Monda V, Villano I, Messina A, Valenzano A, Esposito T, Moscatelli F, Viggiano A, Cibelli G, Chieffi S, Monda M and Messina G (2017) Exercise Modifies the Gut Microbiota with Positive Health Effects. Oxidative Medicine and Cellular Longevity. doi: 10.1155/2017/3831972.

Ohashi Y and Ushida K (2009) Health-beneficial effects of probiotics: Its mode of action. Animal Science Journal 80: 361–371.

Poole L, Hamer M, Wawrzyniak A and Steptoe A (2011) The effects of exercise withdrawal on mood and inflammatory cytokine responses in humans. Stress 14(4): 439–447.

Queipo-Ortuño MI, Seoane LM, Murri M, Pardo M, Gomez-Zumaquero JM, Cardona F, Casanueva F and Tinahones FJ (2013) Gut microbiota composition in male rat models under different nutritional status and physical activity and its association with serum leptin and ghrelin levels. PloS one. 8(5):e65465.

Quigley EMM (2013) Gut bacteria in health and disease. Gastroenterology and Hepatology. 9(9): 560–569.

Rao AV, Bested AC, Beaulne TM, Katzman MA, Lorio C, Berardi JM and Logan AC (2009) A randomized, double blind, placebo controlled pilot study of a probiotic in emotional symptoms of chronic fatigue syndrome. Gut Pathogens 1: 5. doi:10.1186/1757-4749-1-6.

Rhee SH, Pothoulakis C and Mayer EA (2009) Principles and clinical implications of the brain–gutenteric microbiota axis. Nature Reviews Gastroenterology and Hepatology 6: 306–314.

Robles AV and Guarner F (2013) Linking the gut microbiota to human health. British Journal of Nutrition 109: S21–S26.

Steenbergen L, Sellaro R, van Hemert S, Bosch JA and Colzato LS (2015) A randomised controlled trial to test the effect of multispecies probiotics on cognitive reactivity to sad mood. Brain, Behavior and Immunity 48: 258–267.

Strohle A (2009) Physical activity, exercise, depression and anxiety disorders. Journal of Neural Transmission 116: 777–784.

West NP, Pyne DB, Peake JM and Cripps AW (2009) Probiotics, immunity and exercise: a review. Exerc Immunol Rev 15: 107–126.

WHO (2017) Mental disorders. Available from: http://www.who.int/mediacentre/factsheets/fs396/en/ [Accessed 14 December 2017].

Zhu Y, Luo TM, Jobin C and Young HA (2011) Gut microbiota and probiotics in colon tumorigenesis. Cancer Letters 309: 119–127. doi: 10.1016/j.canlet.2011.06.004.

Chapter 4

Impact of Probiotics on Communication between the Brain–Gut

Implications for the Treatment of the Psychological Effects of Digestive Disease States

Mélanie G Gareau[1], Colin Reardon[1], Kim E Barrett[2] and
Philip M Sherman[3,]*

INTRODUCTION

The intestinal microbiota is a complex entity, composed of bacteria, viruses and yeasts. The cumulative genetic material of the microbiota is significant, containing at least ten-times more genetic information than that of the human host, so that it has been described as a virtual "organ within an organ" (Baquero and Nombela, 2012). There is high interpersonal variability, while low intrapersonal variability exists in the microbiota of various body habitats, including the gut, skin and oral cavity and the vagina of women (Costello et al., 2009). A core microbiome (Turnbaugh et al.,

[1] Department of Anatomy, Physiology and Cell Biology, School of Veterinary Medicine, University of California Davis, Davis, CA, USA.
[2] Division of Gastroenterology, School of Medicine, University of California San Diego, La Jolla, CA, USA.
[3] Cell Biology Program, Division of Gastroenterology, Hospital for Sick Children, Toronto, ON, Canada.
* Corresponding author: philip.sherman@sickkids.ca

2009) is shared between individuals and complemented by a variety of phylotypes that differ extensively between individuals, creating a unique and distinguishing microbial fingerprint that is influenced by a variety of factors including host genetics, exposure to antibiotics, and dietary factors including fat content. The microbiome is established starting at birth and its composition is dependent on the route of delivery (vaginal versus cesarean section) and early dietary intake (formula versus breast feeding [including a milk microbiome (Cabrera-Rubio et al., 2012)]). Relative stability of the microbiota is then achieved in early childhood (Isolauri, 2012).

The advent of molecular based sequencing technologies has identified roughly 1,000 different bacterial species in the gastrointestinal tract, mostly in the bacteroides and firmicutes families (Manson et al., 2008). When looked for, Archaea species also appear to be present in the gut microbiota of a proportion of healthy humans. A delicate balance is thought to exist between symbiont and pathobiont organisms in the microbiome that when altered can result in disease (Round and Mazmanian, 2009). Symbiont organisms are composed of a combination of commensal and probiotic organisms thought to be decreased in disease states at the expense of increased colonization by pathobionts.

Changes in the microbiota composition, induced by antibiotic therapy, diet or stress are usually temporary and reversible following removal of the stimulus, although infection with an enteric pathogen can sometimes be associated with ongoing symptoms well beyond removal of the offending infectious agent. For example, treatment with antibiotics and subsequent *Clostridium difficile* infection dramatically shifts the microbiota composition, which undergoes several waves of succession before arriving at a new, different and stable state that is discrete from that present initially (Peterfreund et al., 2012). Maladaptive changes in the composition of the gut microbiota also have been associated with a variety of diseases, ranging from chronic inflammatory bowel disease (IBD) and irritable bowel syndrome (IBS) to obesity and diabetes. In this chapter, we consider the role of probiotics in modulating mood disorders, including anxiety, in the context of intestinal diseases.

Enteric Nerves

The intestinal tract is composed of a single layer of columnar epithelial cells, whose primary functions are to absorb nutrients and to form a barrier between resident microbes in the gut lumen and the host. The location of the epithelium between the microbiota and the underlying lamina propria, which contains nerves, blood vessels, lymphatics, stroma and immune cells, allows for bi-directional host-microbe communication to be established and regulated. The gut is the most highly innervated organ outside the central nervous system (CNS), and contains as many neurons as the peripheral nervous system. This innervation provides a direct link from the gut to the brain, with the vagus nerve prominently mediating various facets of this bi-directional communication.

While the concept of the gut–brain axis is not novel, the idea that the microbiota can regulate either mood or behavior has only recently garnered attention. It has long been known that gut bacteria, including pathogenic *Escherichia coli* strains, respond to nor-epinephrine produced by enteric nerves which promotes the expression of bacterial virulence factors (Lyte et al., 2011). The reverse is also true, with bacteria being capable of inducing neural signals. For instance, administration of *Lactobacillus reuteri*, either live or dead organisms, to healthy rats signals via enteric nerves to reduce constitutive cardio-autonomic responses to colorectal distention (Kamiya et al., 2006). However, these studies did not assess central mechanisms in these rats. The gut microbiota is also required for the development of unique acetylcholine-producing lymphocytes that inhibit innate immune functions (Reardon et al., 2013; Rosas-Ballina et al., 2011). Thus, while it is well-accepted that bacteria can signal locally via enteric nerves and immune mediators, it has only recently been proposed that the gut microbiota may, in fact, signal to the brain.

Probiotics

Probiotics, or beneficial microbes, are defined as organisms added to the diet in such a way as to provide a benefit to the host beyond their inherent nutritional value. Probiotics include, but are not limited to, *Lactobacillus* species, Bifidobacteria and yeasts such as *Saccharomyces boulardii*. Supplementation with these organisms is not a new idea, but the recent increase in popularity in the general population has made organisms more readily available, including commercially in dairy products, breads, creams and drinks.

In recent years, their use has been expanded beyond benefits to the gastrointestinal tract to include brain and mood disorders.

In a rat model of early life stress, maternal separation causes changes in intestinal physiology as well as alterations to the gut–brain axis (Soderholm et al., 2002b), both of which can be normalized by co-treatment with a lactobacillus-preparation containing *L. helveticus* R0052 and *L. rhamnosus* R0011 (Gareau et al., 2007). Similarly, administration of *Bifidobacterium infantis* to rats that previously had been exposed to maternal separation prevented the behavioral, immune and neurotransmitter changes associated with this stress (Desbonnet et al., 2010).

Microbiota-Gut–Brain Axis

The microbiota-gut–brain axis is composed of a bi-directional communication system involving the nervous system (in large part mediated by the vagus nerve), the humoral system (driven by cytokine and chemokine signaling) and the hypothalamic-pituitary-adrenal (HPA)-axis (composed of stress hormones). Studies of the effects of stress on the intestinal tract highlight the role of the luminal microbiota in mediating gut–brain communications. Exposure to stressors can lead to intestinal mucosal barrier dysfunction, thereby allowing microbes access to the underlying lamina propria and both immune and neural-derived cells.

In the lamina propria, microbes are recognized by cells of the immune system, either directly or via enteroendocrine cells, which can activate enteric nerves that signal to the brain. Prolonged, chronic stress leads to changes in the composition of the gut microbiota (Soderholm et al., 2002a), and increased colonization with pathogenic organisms (Bailey et al., 2010). Dysfunction in the microbiota-gut–brain axis is thought to be an underlying cause of functional bowel disorders, including irritable bowel syndrome (IBS). In addition to gastrointestinal symptoms, patients with IBS are more prone to suffer from mood disorders, including anxiety and depression, than the general population and compared to those with underlying organic disease (Lydiard, 2001).

Methods by which the bacteria in the intestinal tract communicate with the brain are emerging as important drivers in establishing normal behavior. Studies using germ-free mice reveal that there are numerous behavioral abnormalities found in the absence of a normal microbiota (Neufeld et al., 2011; Bercik et al., 2011a; Heijtz et al., 2011; Gareau et al., 2011). Germ-free mice display increased motor activity and anxiolytic behavior, with these abnormalities being reversed following microbial colonization in early life (Heijtz et al., 2011). Germ-free mice also demonstrate reduced non-spatial and working memory compared to colonized age-matched controls, which was mediated by changes in hippocampal cFos and brain–derived neurotropic factor (BDNF) expression (Gareau et al., 2011). Similarly, in gut colonized mice administration of an antimicrobial cocktail for 7 days results in an increase in exploratory behavior, which is reversible after removal of the antibiotics (Bercik et al., 2011a).

Behavior and Probiotics

Changes to the intestinal microbiota resulting from an enteric pathogen infection are also associated with the development of changes in normal behavior. Anxiety was observed in mice infected with the murine-specific enteric pathogen *Citrobacter rodentium* 8 hours post-infection, which is prior to the development of a pro-inflammatory response to the infection (Lyte et al., 2006). While the rapid nature of this behavioral response has been taken to indicate that increased anxiety is independent of immune activation, this interpretation is by no means clear or the only biological plausible option. It is important to note that the evidence for lack of immune activation was restricted to serum analysis for levels of interleukin-12, interferon-γ, and tumor necrosis factor-α. While data supporting an alternative hypothesis have not yet been published, it is nonetheless possible that local production of pro-inflammatory cytokines and other immunomodulatory factors that are not reflected in serum assays could have a biological effect on behavior. Furthermore, the 8 h time period after infectious challenge does not allow enough time for colonization of the pathogen in the colon and the ability for the organism to mediate its effects at the site of infection, which is in the distal large intestine. Nevertheless, the suggestion that infection with a bacterial pathogen can rapidly lead to changes in mood has prompted a shift in current understanding of brain–gut microbiota communication and initiated a great deal more interest in mechanistically-oriented research in this area.

Changes in behavior, at least in some cases, can either be prevented or ameliorated with the administration of oral probiotics, including Bifidobacteria and *Lactobacillus* species (Table 1). Memory defects can be ameliorated in mice infected with *C. rodentium* and then exposed to acute psychological stress by the oral pre-treatment

Table 1 Summary of studies demonstrating beneficial effects of probiotics on behavior.

Probiotic/Prebiotic	Beneficial Effect	Reference
Lactobacillus		
L. rhamnosus R0011 and *L. rhamnosus* R0052	Increased non-spatial and working memory in *Citrobacter rodentium* infected mice exposed to acute stress	Gareau et al. 2011
L. rhamnosus JB1	Caused anxiolytic behavior in wild type mice	Bravo et al. 2011
Bifidobacteria		
B. longum NCC3001	Decreased anxiety following *Trichuris muris* infection in mice	Bercik et al. 2011b
B. longum NCC3001	Decreased anxiety-like behavior in mice treated with DSS	Bercik et al. 2011a
Combinations/prebiotics		
L. helveticus R0052 and *B. longum* R0175	Decreased global anxiety and depression scores in healthy volunteers	Messaoudi et al. 2011b
Trans-galactooligosaccharide	Improved anxiety in IBS patients	Silk et al. 2009

of animals with a *Lactobacillus*-containing probiotics cocktail of *L. rhamnosus* R0011 and *L. helveticus* R0052 (Gareau et al., 2010). This intervention not only normalized behavior and the composition of the fecal microbiota, but it also normalized brain physiology with increases in both BDNF and c-fos expression in the hippocampus.

In a mouse model of chronic colitis, caused by dextran sodium sulfate (DSS), administration of *B. longum* strain NCC3001 ameliorated anxiety-like behavior. Anxiety was observed in colitic mice compared to controls, which was then reversed in mice treated with the probiotic strain, but not with a placebo preparation (Bercik et al., 2011b). Similarly, mice infected with a parasite, *Trichuris muris*, developed anxiety, which could be prevented by treatment with the probiotic *B. longum* NCC3001, but not *L. rhamnosus* NCC4007 (Bercik et al., 2010). In normal wild-type mice, administration of *L. rhamnosus* JB-1 demonstrated anxiolytic effects in behavior, compared to sham fed controls and was mediated by the GABA-nergic system (Bravo et al., 2011). Furthermore, treatment with probiotics also prevented stress-induced increases in serum corticosterone, suggesting that probiotics provide a beneficial effect on behavior under both baseline and stress conditions (Bravo et al., 2011). This study was the first to demonstrate an effect of probiotics in regulating normal, physiological host responses.

Intestinal inflammation can lead to the development of anxiety in mice, which can be prevented by daily treatment with probiotic organisms. Therefore, not only do probiotics normalize the local environment in the intestinal tract by modulating the composition and functions of the gut microbiota, but they also can normalize brain physiology and behavior. Proper selection of probiotic organisms utilized for specific benefits is therefore important and it remains to be determined by which exact underlying mechanisms these changes are mediated.

In human studies, psychological effects of administration of a *Lactobacillus/* Bifidobacteria-containing mixture (*L. rhamnosus* R0052 and *B. longum* R0175) to healthy volunteers were determined. Following 30 days of treatment, a double-blind, placebo-controlled, randomized trial revealed a decrease in global scores for hospital anxiety and depression scale, alleviating psychological distress (Messaoudi et al., 2011a; Messaoudi et al., 2011b). In patients with IBS, a parallel crossover trial revealed an improvement in both severity of bowel symptoms score and anxiety score following 12 weeks of daily oral administration of a prebiotic, trans-galactooligosaccharide (Silk et al., 2009). This effect was thought to be produced by ability of the prebiotic to serve as a fermentation substrate, thereby increasing colonic Bifidobacteria concentrations.

While probiotics are now considered as a possible effective strategy for preventing alterations in the components of the gut–brain axis, recent evidence suggests that the use of treatment regimens may also provide beneficial effects. In a chronic DSS-induced colitis model, mice developed anxiety-like behavior (Bercik et al., 2011b). Administration of *B. longum* NCC3001 following completion of two cycles of DSS had an anxiolytic effect, highlighting that pre-treatment is not an absolute prerequisite for the beneficial effects of probiotics. Using the *C. rodentium* model, we showed that co-treatment or even early post-infection administration of the probiotics *L. rhamnosus* R0011 and *L. helveticus* R0052 could prevent enteric infection-induced gut inflammation and changes in intestinal physiology (Rodrigues et al., 2012). While behavior was not assessed in these mice, the findings do suggest that probiotics can serve as a potential therapeutic option to treat established microbiome-gut–brain axis mediated disorders.

In addition to probiotics, other dietary changes can also alter the composition of the gut microbiota with beneficial impacts on brain functions. For instance, mouse chow supplemented with 50% lean ground beef protein improved cognitive parameters compared to normal rodent chow, including working and reference memory, in the context of a more diverse gut microbiota composition (Li et al., 2009). Therefore, dietary manipulations may provide an alternative method of changing the microbiota in certain subsets of immune compromised patients, where concerns may arise with the use of live organisms.

Mood Disorders in GI Disease

Changes in behavior are increasingly recognized as a factor common to many diseases in humans, including gastrointestinal disorders. Psycho-neuro-endocrine-immune modulation appears to be involved in the pathogenesis of IBD, which occurs via changes in the gut–brain-microbiota axis (Bonaz and Bernstein, 2013). Patients with inflammatory bowel diseases (Crohn's disease and ulcerative colitis) and irritable bowel syndrome (IBS) are prone to develop concurrent mood disorders, including anxiety and depression (Goodhand et al., 2012; Lydiard, 2001), which are more prevalent under conditions of perceived stress (Goodhand et al., 2012). An increased presence of anxiety and depression is associated with decreased quality-of-life in both IBD and IBS patients (Gray et al., 2011). Moreover, co-morbid depression was associated with increased disease activity in patients with IBD (Faust et al., 2012). Stress is associated with increased mucosal inflammation in both patients and in animal models of IBD (Mawdsley and Rampton, 2005; Mawdsley and Rampton, 2006). Furthermore, mood disorders are associated with decreased compliance with prescribed treatments (Gray et al., 2012), likely contributing to decreased maintenance of disease remission. The presence of these mood disorders also can lead to the development of secondary functional GI diseases requiring additional therapeutic interventions and complicating treatment regimens (Figure 1). Behavioral interventions in patients with IBD are associated with an increase in the duration of remission of disease activity (Keefer et al., 2011).

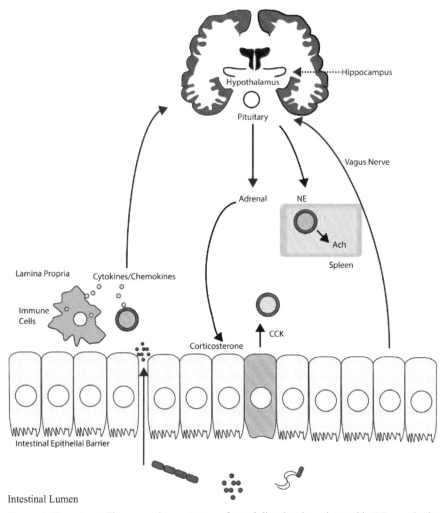

Figure 1   Flow chart. The concomitant presence of mood disorders in patients with IBD may lead to the development of secondary functional gastrointestinal diseases (FGID) that can complicate treatment regimens and decrease compliance. Interruption of this cycle with probiotics could serve to ameliorate the burden of disease and improve daily quality-of-life for affected patients.

Mechanisms by Which Probiotics Regulate Anxiety

The numerous connections existing between the gut and the brain provide multiple possible mechanisms through which probiotics could regulate the brain, including the vagus nerve (Figure 2).

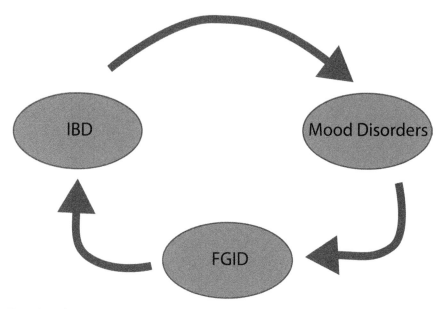

Figure 2 Brain–gut-microbiota axis pathways. Multiple potential pathways exist for communications between the brain and the gut. The hypothalamus-pituitary-adrenal (HPA)-axis results in corticosterone release, which can signal via immune cells or epithelial cells to affect mucosal epithelial barrier function. Feedback inhibition of the HPA-axis occurs at the level of both the hypothalamus and hippocampus. An increase in gut permeability, in patients with IBD or IBS, can result in the translocation of microbes into the underlying lamina propria, which then activates immune cells to produce pro-inflammatory cytokines. Vagal efferent signals terminating in the celiac ganglion induce the release of nor-epinephrine (NE) from splenic neurons. The neurotransmitter acts on a specific population of CD4+ T-cells, through beta-adrenergic receptors, to induce the release of acetylcholine (Ach). Ach is also released from B-cells following stimulation with cholecystokinin (CCK), the source of which is enteroendocrine cells contained in the intestinal tract.

The vagus nerve

A role for the vagus nerve in mediating intestinal microbiota-mediated changes in the brain and behavior has been suggested in some studies, but not in others. The integrity of the vagus nerve was important in mediating the beneficial effects of *B. longum* administration on anxiety in DSS-induced colitis (Bercik et al., 2011b). In wild-type mice treated with *L. rhamnosus*, a role for the vagus nerve was also observed in mediating GABA-receptor signaling and stress-induced anxiety-related behavior (Bravo et al., 2011). In contrast, sub-diaphragmatic vagotomy did not prevent the beneficial effect on anxiety observed following administration of *B. longum* in the context of infection with *T. muris*, excluding a role for the vagus in this model (Bercik et al., 2010). It is possible that the role of the vagus nerve on mediating the effects of probiotics on brain function depends on both the specific model of intestinal inflammation employed and on the strain of probiotic organism studied.

One aspect that has not been addressed by studies published to date relates to the site of innervation versus the location of the beneficial effect being sought. For instance, the vagus nerve does not innervate the distal colon, which is the most common site for colonization by probiotics and for injury and inflammation in many models of colitis. This could account for a lack of beneficial effect on behavior of probiotics in some models of gut injury. Perhaps a role for pelvic splanchnic innervation should be sought in future research studies evaluating the role of probiotics colonizing the gut on outcomes in the central nervous system.

HPA-axis

Programming of the HPA-axis occurs early in life and is closely shaped by dam-pup interactions in rats. Activation of the HPA-axis is associated with stress-induced changes in intestinal function. Dysregulation of the HPA-axis, as a result of exposure to early life stress via neonatal maternal separation, is associated with long-lasting maladaptive stress responses. These changes lead to both mucosal barrier dysfunction (Gareau et al., 2006) and alterations in immune regulation (Shanks et al., 2000). In addition to barrier dysfunction, early life stress also leads to depression (Soderholm et al., 2002b; Varghese et al., 2006), anxiety-like behavior (Soderholm et al., 2002b), changes in the intestinal microbiota (O'Mahony et al., 2009) and the development of more severe colitis than in non-stressed controls (Varghese et al., 2006; Barreau et al., 2004), which can be treated with anti-depressants (Varghese et al., 2006). Interestingly, the beneficial effects of anti-depressants in maternal separation were mediated by the vagus nerve, as indicated by the absence of improvement in colonic inflammation following subdiaphragmic vagotomy (Ghia et al., 2008).

Exposure to either physical or psychological stress is associated with changes in intestinal physiology. Acute stress is associated with HPA-axis activation and mucosal barrier dysfunction, whereas chronic stress is associated with more pronounced changes including mucosal inflammation and changes to the composition and function of the gut microbiota (Soderholm et al., 2002a; Saunders et al., 1994). Changes in intestinal permeability produced by stress provides translocating intact and viable bacteria access to the underlying lamina propria, which then results in activation of the local mucosal immune system (Bailey et al., 2006).

The gut microbiota plays an important role in the development of the HPA-axis, with germ-free mice having an increase in baseline serum corticosterone levels (Sudo et al., 2004). Administration of probiotics during exposure to early life stress can prevent the deleterious effects on HPA-axis and gut physiology in both neonatal and adult animals (Gareau et al., 2007). Exposure to a prolonged, severe physical restraint stressor changes the composition of the microbiota and increases colonization with *C. rodentium* (Bailey et al., 2010). Similarly, exposure to psychological stress, using a model of social disruption, caused changes in the gut microbiota that resulted in increased levels of circulating pro-inflammatory cytokines, as demonstrated by abrogation of inflammatory mediators when mice were treated with antibiotics (Bailey et al., 2011). Taken together, these findings indicate that signaling via the

HPA-axis provides a means of communication between probiotics colonizing the gut epithelia and the brain.

Immune system

Underlying the epithelial mucosa is a dense network of immune cells, which constantly survey for the presence of potentially noxious antigens. Circulating pro-inflammatory cytokines produced when the immune system is exposed to either bacteria or bacterial-derived products, perhaps as a result of a breach in the integrity of the epithelial barrier, contributes to behavioral signaling in the brain. Maternal separation, for example, causes colonic inflammation in both neonatal (Gareau et al., 2006) and adult (Barreau et al., 2004) rats, as well as increased colonic Toll-like receptor (TLR) expression (including TLR3, TLR4 and TLR5) (McKernan et al., 2009), suggesting a local micro-environment where immune cell signaling is involved. Using a chronic mild stress model of depression in rats, administration of a monoclonal antibody against TNFα decreased depression and anxiety-like behavior, compared to placebo (Karson et al., 2012). While it is clear that a relationship exists between stress, inflammation, the gut microbiota and behavior, the exact pathways by which microbes mediate changes in behavior are still being unraveled.

Conclusions

Roles for the resident gut microbiota and probiotics in alleviating mood disorders, including anxiety, are increasingly being recognized, especially in the settings of gastrointestinal diseases such as IBS and IBD. Relevant animal models indicate a number of pathways by which this communication may be regulated. Stress and mood disorders enhance clinical symptoms and increase underlying disease severity in patients with IBD. Critical evaluation of the use of probiotics as a means to limit the development of anxiety and depression in IBD and IBS is therefore warranted. Finding the right probiotic strain for use in the appropriate setting could well prove to have a clinically relevant effect in limiting mood disorders in patients with chronic disease and altered composition and function of their gut microbiota.

References

Bailey MT, Engler H and Sheridan JF (2006) Stress induces the translocation of cutaneous and gastrointestinal microflora to secondary lymphoid organs of C57BL/6 mice. Journal of Neuroimmunology 171: 29–37.

Bailey MT, Dowd SE, Parry NM, Galley JP, Schauer DB and Lyte M (2010) Stressor exposure disrupts commensal microbial populations in the intestines and leads to increased colonization by Citrobacter rodentium. Infection and Immunity 78: 1509–1519.

Bailey MT, Dowd SE, Galley JD, Hufnagle AR, Allen RG and Lyte M (2011) Exposure to a social stressor alters the structure of the intestinal microbiota: implications for stressor-induced immunomodulation. Brain, Behavior, and Immunity 25: 397–407.

Baquero F and Nombela C (2012) The microbiome as a human organ. Clinical Microbiology and Infection 18 Suppl 4: 2–4.

Barreau F, Ferrier L, Fioramonti J and Bueno L (2004) Neonatal maternal deprivation triggers long term alterations in colonic epithelial barrier and mucosal immunity in rats. Gut 53: 501–506.

Bercik P, Verdu EF, Foster JA, Marci J, Potter M, Huang x, Mallinowski P, Jackson W, Blennerhassett P, Neufeld KA, Lu J, Khan WI, Corthesy-Theulaz I, Cherbut C, Bergonzelli GE and Collins SM (2010) Chronic gastrointestinal inflammation induces anxiety-like behavior and alters central nervous system biochemistry in mice. Gastroenterology 139: 2102–2112 e2101.

Bercik P, Denou E, Collins J, Jackson W, Lu J, Jury J, Deng Y, Blennerhassett PA, Marci J, McCoy KD, Verdu EF and collins SM (2011a) The intestinal microbiota affect central levels of brain-derived neurotropic factor and behavior in mice. Gastroenterology 141: 599–609 e593.

Bercik P, Park AJ, Sinclair D, Khoshdel A, Lu J, Huang X, Deng Y, Blennerhassett PA, Fahenstock M, Moine D, Berger B, Huizinga JD, Kunze W, Mclean PG, Bergonzelli GE, Collins SM and Verdu EF (2011b) The anxiolytic effect of Bifidobacterium longum NCC3001 involves vagal pathways for gut–brain communication. Neurogastroenterology and Motility 23: 1132–1139.

Bonaz BL and Bernstein CN (2013) Brain-gut interactions in inflammatory bowel disease. Gastroenterology 144: 36–49.

Bravo JA, Forsythe P, Chew MV, Escaravage E, Savignac HM, Dinan TG, Bienenstock J and Cryan JF (2011) Ingestion of Lactobacillus strain regulates emotional behavior and central GABA receptor expression in a mouse via the vagus nerve. Proceedings of the National Academy of Sciences of the United States of America 108: 16050–16055.

Cabrera-Rubio R, Collado MC, Laitinen K, Salminen S, Isolauri E and Mira A (2012) The human milk microbiome changes over lactation and is shaped by maternal weight and mode of delivery. Am J Clinical Nutrition 96: 544–551.

Costello EK, Lauber CL, Hamady M, Fierer N, Gordon JI and Knight R (2009) Bacterial community variation in human body habitats across space and time. Science 326: 1694–1697.

Desbonnet L, Garrett L, Clarke G, Kiely B, Cryan JF and Dinan TG (2010) Effects of the probiotic Bifidobacterium infantis in the maternal separation model of depression. Neuroscience 170: 1179–1188.

Faust AH, Halpern LF, Danoff-Burg S and Cross RK (2012) Psychosocial factors contributing to inflammatory bowel disease activity and health-related quality of life. Clinical Gastroenterology and Hepatology (N Y) 8: 173–181.

Gareau MG, Jury J, Yang PC, MacQueen G and Perdue MH (2006) Neonatal maternal separation causes colonic dysfunction in rat pups including impaired host resistance. Pediatric Research 59: 83–88.

Gareau MG, Jury J, MacQueen G, Sherman PM and Perdue MH (2007) Probiotic treatment of rat pups normalises corticosterone release and ameliorates colonic dysfunction induced by maternal separation. Gut 56: 1522–1528.

Gareau MG, Wine E, Reardon C and Sherman PM (2010) Probiotics prevent death caused by Citrobacter rodentium infection in neonatal mice. Journal of Infectious Diseases 201: 81–91.

Gareau MG, Wine E, Rodrigues DM, Cjoo JH, Whary MT, Philpott DJ, MacQueen G and Sherman PM (2011) Bacterial infection causes stress-induced memory dysfunction in mice. Gut 60: 307–317.

Ghia JE, Blennerhassett P and Collins SM (2008) Impaired parasympathetic function increases susceptibility to inflammatory bowel disease in a mouse model of depression. Journal of Clinical Investigation 118: 2209–2218.

Goodhand JR, Wahed M, Mawdsley JE, Farmer AD, Aziz Q and Rampton DS (2012) Mood disorders in inflammatory bowel disease: Relation to diagnosis, disease activity, perceived stress, and other factors. Inflammatory Bowel Diseases.

Gray WN, Denson LA, Baldassano RN and Hommel KA (2011) Disease activity, behavioral dysfunction, and health-related quality of life in adolescents with inflammatory bowel disease. Inflammatory Bowel Diseases 17: 1581–1586.

Gray WN, Denson LA, Baldassano RN and Hommel KA (2012) Treatment adherence in adolescents with inflammatory bowel disease: the collective impact of barriers to adherence and anxiety/depressive symptoms. Journal of Pediatric Psychology 37: 282–291.

Heijtz RD, Wang S, Anuar F, Quian Y, Bjorkholm B, Samuelsson A, Hibberd ML, Fossberg H and Pettersson S (2011) Normal gut microbiota modulates brain development and behavior. Proceedings of the National Academy of Sciences of the United States of America 108: 3047–3052.

Isolauri E (2012) Development of healthy gut microbiota early in life. J Paediatr Child Health 48 Suppl 3: 1–6.

Kamiya T, Wang L, Forsythe P, Goettsche G, Mao Y, Wang Y, Tongas G and Bienenstock J (2006) Inhibitory effects of Lactobacillus reuteri on visceral pain induced by colorectal distension in Sprague-Dawley rats. Gut 55: 191–196.

Karson A, Demirtas T, Bayramgurler D, Balci F and Utkan T (2012) Chronic administration of infliximab (TNF-Alpha Inhibitor) decreases depression and anxiety-like behaviour in rat model of chronic mild stress. Basic & Clinical Pharmacology & Toxicology.

Keefer L, Kiebles JL, Martinovich Z, Cohen E, VanDenburg A and Barrett TA (2011) Behavioral interventions may prolong remission in patients with inflammatory bowel disease. Behaviour Research and Therapy 49: 145–150.

Li W, Dowd SE, Scurlock B, Acosta-Martinez V and Lyte M (2009) Memory and learning behavior in mice is temporally associated with diet-induced alterations in gut bacteria. Physiology & Behavior 96: 557–567.

Lydiard RB (2001) Irritable bowel syndrome, anxiety, and depression: what are the links? The Journal of Clinical Psychiatry 62 Suppl 8: 38–45.

Lyte M, Li W, Opitz N, Gaykema RP and Goehler LE (2006) Induction of anxiety-like behavior in mice during the initial stages of infection with the agent of murine colonic hyperplasia Citrobacter rodentium. Physiology & Behavior 89: 350–357.

Lyte M, Vulchanova L and Brown DR (2011) Stress at the intestinal surface: catecholamines and mucosa-bacteria interactions. Cell and Tissue Research 343: 23–32.

Manson JM, Rauch M and Gilmore MS (2008) The commensal microbiology of the gastrointestinal tract. Advances in Experimental Medicine and Biology 635: 15–28.

Mawdsley JE and Rampton DS (2005) Psychological stress in IBD: new insights into pathogenic and therapeutic implications. Gut 54: 1481–1491.

Mawdsley JE and Rampton DS (2006) The role of psychological stress in inflammatory bowel disease. Neuroimmunomodulation 13: 327–336.

McKernan DP, Nolan A and Brint EK (2009) Toll-like receptor mRNA expression is selectively increased in the colonic mucosa of two animal models relevant to irritable bowel syndrome. PLoS One 4: e8226.

Messaoudi M, Lalonde R, Violle N, Javelot H, Desdor D, Nejdi A, Bisson JF, Rouget C, Pichelin M and Cazaubiel JM (2011a) Assessment of psychotropic-like properties of a probiotic formulation (Lactobacillus helveticus R0052 and Bifidobacterium longum R0175) in rats and human subjects. British Journal of Nutrition 105: 755–764.

Messaoudi M, Violle N, Bisson JF, Dessor D, Javelot H and Rouget C (2011b) Beneficial psychological effects of a probiotic formulation (Lactobacillus helveticus R0052 and Bifidobacterium longum R0175) in healthy human volunteers. Gut Microbes 2: 256–261.

Neufeld KM, Kang N, Bienenstock J and Foster JA (2011) Reduced anxiety-like behavior and central neurochemical change in germ-free mice. Neurogastroenterology and Motility: The Official Journal of the European Gastrointestinal Motility Society 23: 255–264, e119.

O'Mahony SM, Marchesi JR, Scully P, Coldling C, Ceolho AM, Quigley EM, Cryan JF and Dinan TG (2009) Early life stress alters behavior, immunity, and microbiota in rats: implications for irritable bowel syndrome and psychiatric illnesses. Biological Psychiatry 65: 263–267.

Peterfreund GL, Vandivier LE, Sinha R, Marozsan AJ, Olson WC, Zhu J and Bushman FD (2012) Succession in the gut microbiome following antibiotic and antibody therapies for Clostridium difficile. PLoS One 7: e46966.

Reardon C, Duncan GS, Brustle A, Brenner D, Tusche MW, Olofsson PS, Rosa-Ballina M, Tracey KJ and Mak TW (2013) Lymphocyte-derived ACh regulates local innate but not adaptive immunity. Proceedings of the National Academy of Sciences of the United States of America.

Rodrigues DM, Sousa AJ, Johnson-Henry KC, Sherman PM and Gareau MG (2012) Probiotics are effective for the prevention and treatment of Citrobacter rodentium-induced colitis in mice. The Journal of Infectious Diseases 206: 99–109.

Rosas-Ballina M, Olofsson PS, Ochani M, Valdes-Ferrer SI, Levine YA, Reardon C, Tusche MW, Pavlov VA, Andersson U, Charan S, Mak TW and Tracey KJ (2011) Acetylcholine-synthesizing T cells relay neural signals in a vagus nerve circuit. Science 334: 98–101.

Round JL and Mazmanian SK (2009) The gut microbiota shapes intestinal immune responses during health and disease. Nature Reviews Immunology 9: 313–323.

Saunders PR, Kosecka U, McKay DM and Perdue MH (1994) Acute stressors stimulate ion secretion and increase epithelial permeability in rat intestine. American Journal of Physiology-Gastrointestinal and Liver Physiology 30: G794–G799.

Shanks N, Windle RJ, Perks PA, Harbuz MS, Jessop DS, Ingram CD and Lightman SL (2000) Early-life exposure to endotoxin alters hypothalamic-pituitary-adrenal function and predisposition to inflammation. Proceedings of the National Academy of Sciences of the United States of America 97: 5645–5650.

Silk DB, Davis A, Vulevic J, Tzortzis G and Gibson GR (2009) Clinical trial: the effects of a trans-galactooligosaccharide prebiotic on faecal microbiota and symptoms in irritable bowel syndrome. Alimentary Pharmacology & Therapeutics 29: 508–518.

Soderholm JD, Yang PC, Ceponis P, Vohra A, Riddell R, Sherman PM and Perdue MH (2002a) Chronic stress induces mast cell-dependent bacterial adherence and initiates mucosal inflammation in rat intestine. Gastroenterology 123: 1099–1108.

Soderholm JD, Yates DA, Gareau MG, Yang PC, MacQueen G and Perdue MH (2002b) Neonatal maternal separation predisposes adult rats to colonic barrier dysfunction in response to mild stress. American Journal of Physiology-Gastrointestinal and Liver Physiology 283: G1257–1263.

Sudo N, Chida Y, Aiba Y, Sonoda J, Oyama N, Yu XN, Kubo C and Koga Y (2004) Postnatal microbial colonization programs the hypothalamic-pituitary-adrenal system for stress response in mice. The Journal of Physiology while 558: 263–275.

Turnbaugh PJ, Hamady M, Yatsunenko T, Cantrel BL, Duncan A, Ley RE, Sogin ML, Jones WJ, Roe BA, Affourtit JP, Egholm M, Henrissat B, Heath AC, Knight R and Gordon JI (2009) A core gut microbiome in obese and lean twins. Nature 457: 480–484.

Varghese AK, Verdu EF, Bercik P, Khan WI, Blennerhassett PA, Szectman H and Collins SM (2006) Antidepressants attenuate increased susceptibility to colitis in a murine model of depression. Gastroenterology 130: 1743–1753.

Chapter 5

Probiotics and their Effect on Maternal and Neonatal Health

Caroline J Hollins Martin[1,]* and *Colin R Martin*[2]

INTRODUCTION

Probiotics are living microorganisms which when dispensed in sufficient quantities are claimed to bestow benefits in terms of health on the host (WHO, 2001). The word probiotic is a composite of two Greek expressions: *pro* which means endorsement of and *biotic* denotes life (Hamilton-Miller et al., 2003). In essence, the word probiotic symbolises well-being and life, through selectively stimulating growth and activity of intestinal bacteria that contribute to health and well-being. It is important for health care professionals not to dismiss the positive effects of probiotics for childbearing women during pregnancy, since the latest research reports that live active cultures of friendly bacterias can facilitate prevention of a variety of ailments. Hence, maternity care professionals (e.g., midwives, obstetricians, health visitors, general practitioners) need to know how to provide evidence-based information about the advantages and disadvantages of probiotic consumption, across pregnancy, birth, postnatal and infancy (see Figure 1). The key message for maternity health care professionals is that probiotics and prebiotics from natural food sources and

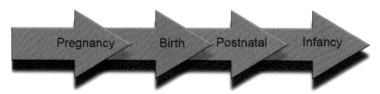

Figure 1 The continuum of pregnancy, birth, postnatal and infancy.

[1] Edinburgh Napier University, Edinburgh, Scotland, UK.
[2] Buckinghamshire New University, Middlesex, England, UK.
* Corresponding author: C.HollinsMartin@napier.ac.uk

supplements are considered safe for childbearing women to consume as long as the manufacturers' guidelines are followed. The aim of taking probiotics is to modify GI tract flora and replace harmful microbes with useful microbes. Probiotics are live microorganisms that bear similarity to those naturally present in the human GI system, with milk fermented with lactic-acid bacteria fermenting lactose and lowering the GI pH. For the majority, mention of probiotics conjures up images of yoghurt, which does not appeal to everyone, especially when troubled with morning sickness during pregnancy. The purpose of this chapter is to provide information for maternity care professionals about what is known and not known about probiotics. Contents of discussion will address:

- What probiotics are.
- Examples of beneficial probiotic organisms.
- What food products contain probiotics.
- Probiotic effect upon the systems in childbearing women and neonates.

What are Probiotics?

The World Health Organization (WHO, 2001) defines a probiotic as any living microorganism that produces a health benefit when ingested. As such, probiotic organisms are live bacteria considered to be advantageous due to the lactic acid produced, which affords benefits to the host in terms of preventing pathogenic bacterial growth. Active live cultures of specific microbes are commonly added to yoghurts or sold in tablet or capsule form.

Probiotics were first discovered by a male Russian microbiologist called Elie Metchnikoff who won the Nobel Peace Prize for his efforts. Metchnikoff's research initiated ongoing debates about advantages and disadvantages of whether or not humans should consume probiotics. According to Sanders (2003) key features of probiotics include:

- They must be alive (although it is acknowledged that dead cells in some instances have advantage).
- Must convey specified benefits to the host.
- May be administered in foods, tablet/capsule form or given rectally.
- Specified strains impact upon named microbes of a known composition.

Probiotics are a preparation containing viable, defined microorganisms in sufficient numbers to alter microflora through implantation or colonization in a compartment of the host, thus exerting beneficial health effects on the host (Havenaar and Huis In't Veld, 1992; Schrezenmeir and de Vrese, 2001). According to Roberfroid (2007) probiotics are a dietary carbohydrate that is resistant to:

- Gastric acidity.
- Hydrolysis by mammalian enzymes.
- Gastro Intestinal (GI) absorption.
- Fermentation by intestinal microflora.

In contrast to probiotics, prebiotics are selectively fermented ingredients that allow specific changes to take place in composition and activity of the gastrointestinal microflora (Roberfroid, 2007). Essentially, prebiotics are nondigestible food ingredients that beneficially affect the host by selectively stimulating growth and activity of one or a limited number of bacteria in the colon and by doing so improve host health.

Due to an absence of sufficient research about probiotic use in pregnancy, at present there is no recommended daily allowance. Despite a dearth of information and an invitation for future research, there are no reports of pregnant women or foetus's having encountered harm from taking probiotics (Dugoua et al., 2009; Osborn and Sinn, 2007). A question that may be asked by childbearing women of a maternity care expert is, whether or not probiotics are beneficial to take during pregnancy? The majority of probiotics that can be purchased off the shelves of holistic health shops, chemists and supermarkets are of questionable quality, quite simply because not enough research has been carried out to provide evidence of benefits of specific probiotic strains and appropriate dosages in relation to named disorders and their prevention or improvement. For many of the espoused benefits from taking probiotics, there remains a dearth of proof about their effectiveness in relation to named variables.

Examples of Beneficial Probiotic Organisms

Probiotics added to products by manufacturers are required to survive the hostile acid and bile of the upper GI tract, with several probiotic strains investigated to ascertain health benefits (Reid et al., 2004). For example, *Lactobacillus rhamnosus*, *Lactobacillus reuteri* and *Saccharomyces boulardii*.

Lactobacillus rhamnosus

Lactobacillus rhamnosus is occasionally used in yoghurts and yoghurt drinks. It was originally isolated in 1983 from the GI tract of a healthy human by Gorbach and Goldin. *Lactobacillus rhamnosus* survives the acid and bile of the human GI tract and inhibits pathogen growth through release of acids, bacteriocins and hydrogen peroxide. As such, it can be used to prevent and treat diarrhea (Canaani et al., 2007; Guandalini et al., 2000; Österlund et al., 2007), respiratory infections (Hatakka et al., 2001; Hojsak et al., 2009), atopic dermatitis (mixed reviews) (Boyle et al., 2009; Kalliomäki et al., 2001, 2007) and GI tract vancomycin resistant enterococcus (Manley et al., 2007).

Lactobacillus reuteri

Lactobacillus reuteri is bacteria that naturally inhabits the GI tract of humans and was originally identified by Kandler et al. in 1980. *Lactobacillus reuteri* produces reuterin in the GI tract, which inhibits growth of *Escherichia coli* (Cleusix et al., 2008). Oral intake increases secretion of *Lactobacillus reuteri* in breast milk (Sinkiewicz and Nordström, 2005), which is then transferred into the GI tract of breastfeeding infants (Abrahamsson et al., 2005), thus affording them infection protection. Further evidence supports that *Lactobacillus reuteri* partially eradicates *Helicobacter Pylori*, which causes peptic ulcers (Imase et al., 2007), *Streptococcus Mutans* which causes tooth decay (Nikawa et al., 2004) and is effective at alleviating gingivitis (Krasse et al., 2006). In addition, adults who take probiotics containing *Lactobacillus reuteri* have been recorded to have 50% less sick episodes (Tubelius, 2005).

Saccharomyces boulardii

*Saccharomyces boulardii i*s a tropical strain of yeast that was isolated from lychee and mangosteen fruit in 1923 by the French scientist Henri Boulard. So far, two studies have identified significant reduction in symptoms of acute gastroenteritis in children (Castagliuolo et al., 1999; Saint-Marc et al., 1995). To be effective, infants less than 3 months old should be given half a 250 mg capsule or sachet 2 times a day for 5 days. In a placebo controlled prospective RCT, Gedek (1999) found a significant reduction in diarrhoea symptoms in adults who took 250 mg of *Saccharomyces boulardii* 2 times a day for 5 days. *Saccharomyces boulardii* has also been shown to increase emission of the Immunoglobulin A(IgA) in the small intestines of rats (Buts et al., 1990). Taking oral gelatin capsules containing dried *L. rhamnosus GR-1* and *L. reuteri RC-14* decrease the chances of women developing bacterial vaginosis through maintenance of regular lactobacilli vaginal flora (Reid et al., 2001, 2003, 2008). In research studies that have utilized animals as participants, strains were found to improve health of female rats and their newborn (Anukam et al., 2005). Lactobacilli also play a part in prevention of colonization by group *B. streptococci* of the vagina, which can cause rigorous disease, potential blindness and mortality in neonates (Acikgoz et al., 2005).

What Food Products contain Probiotics?

A Colony Forming Unit (CFU) is the microbiological term to quantify the amount of viable bacteria in a produce. The CFU informs us how much probiotic a particular food product contains and what in fact will be available for use by the human body. The gastroenterologist Challa (2012) states that it is not possible to quantify precise amounts of probiotics because these live microorganisms (in most cases bacteria) are so similar to those naturally found in the GI tract. Also known as friendly or good bacteria, probiotics are the cornerstone of a potentially successful health program because they restore equilibrium between friendly and injurious bacteria in the GI tract, with a balance critical for health of the human body. Probiotics are associated with treating many human conditions. Examples of these include Irritable Bowel Syndrome (IBS), forms of cancer, allergies, eczema and the effects of aging. Challa (2012) explains how taking the right probiotics in the form of food or food supplements incurs health benefits. One method of achieving advantage is to create recipes that infuse probiotics into the childbearing women's diet. To view examples of content of probiotic food products (see Table 1):

Table 1 Examples of types of food products that infuse probiotics into diet and the potential benefits.

Recipes	Potential benefits
Smoothies and juices Smoothie and juice recipes that utilise yoghurt as the chief constituent mixed with fresh fruits and liquidised. Examples include, watermelon and yoghurt with crushed ice, carrot and yoghurt smoothie, banana peanut and yoghurt smoothie.	In addition to health advantages of probiotics the childbearing woman receives vitamins from fruit components.
Soups and salad Soup and salad recipes that utilize yoghurt as one of the main dressing ingredients. Examples include potatoe salad with yoghurt dressing or cucumber and yoghurt and vitamins from the fruit and vegetables.	Provides a solid combination of health advantages of probiotics from the yoghurt.
Main meals Serve main meals with yoghurt added. For example, spaghetti with tomato yoghurt, roast chicken yoghurt, tuna and hard-boiled egg yoghurt fillings for sandwiches and pitta pockets, curries with mint yoghurt and cucumber dressing.	Produces a tasty vitamin and probiotic rich meal.
Yoghurt and fruit puddings Add yoghurt to cakes instead of cream or ice cream. For example, banana yoghurt cake, fresh pancakes with fruit and yoghurt, cheese cake with yoghurt, cookies with yoghurt, fruit yoghurt mousse.	Reduces calorie intake and produces a tasty vitamin and probiotic rich sweet.

In a non-pharmaceutical capacity, probiotic rich recipes help (Challa, 2012):

- Improve the health of the childbearing woman's GI tract.
- Alleviate allergies and asthma.
- Facilitate the reproductive and urinary tract.
- Bolster the immune system against disease.
- Enhance weight loss.

To compliment diet, supplements that contain probiotic bacteria can be purchased without prescription in the form of capsules, tablets and powders. These can be bought in most natural health food shops. Some would argue that it is unnecessary to purchase such supplements, quite simply because so many food products naturally contain probiotics. In addition, there are manufacturers who make, advertise and sell food products supplemented with probiotics. Food products which contain added probiotics include:

- Live yoghurts.
- Yoghurt drinks.
- Cheese.
- Fermented and unfermented milk.
- Sour cream.
- Kifir which is a fermented milk drink.

- Miso and tempeh made from fermented soya beans.
- Some juices.
- Soya drinks.

Many of these products may already be part of the childbearing woman's daily diet. Within these food products, the probiotic bacteria may comprise its original content or else be added by a manufacturer. Some consider that adding probiotics to food products is an unnecessary task, since many already have *prebiotics* as part of their constitution. *Prebiotics* that facilitate growth of friendly bacteria are carbohydrates called Fructo Oligo Saccharides (FOS). FOS carbohydrates naturally occur in:

- Artichokes
- Asparagus
- Bananas
- Barley
- Chicory
- Garlic
- Oats
- Onions
- Soya beans

Prebiotic FOS carbohydrates can also be purchased as supplements. Particular dynamics influence survival of probiotics in food products and they are considered during the manufacturing process. These include:

- Physiological state of the added probiotic in the food.
- Physiochemical conditions of food processing.
- Physical conditions of product storage, e.g., temperature and chemical composition.
- Nutrients, oxygen or pH interactions with other product components that are inhibitory or protective.

Probiotic Effect upon the Systems in Childbearing Women and Neonates

Of particular interest is addressing what to date is known about probiotics and their effects upon the systems of the body.

The Gastro Intestinal (GI) Tract

Probiotics play a key role in regulation and maintenance of the biochemical balance of the GI tract through obstructing growth of toxin producing bacteria and alleviating intestinal inflammatory disease (Mach, 2006) and pathogen-induced diarrhoea (Yan and Polk, 2006).

Sometimes probiotics are prescribed in the form of fecal material taken from a healthy donor, which are then inserted in suppository form into a person who has inflammatory bowel disease and is infected with Clostridium Difficile (Bakken et al., 2011; Borody et al., 2011). Some strains of Lactic Acid Bacteria (LAB) displace pathogenic microorganisms through competitive cohabitation, and as such are considered effective towards treating acute diarrhea and in particular rotovirus infections in infants, children and adults (Reid et al. 2003; Ouwehand, 2002). A few manufactured probiotic products are associated with positive outcomes. For example, *Lactobacillus rhamnosus GG (ConAgra), B. lactis BB12* with *Lactobacillus acidophilus La5*, and *Lactobacillus reuteri SD2112*, all of which are reported to effectively treat diarrhea (Guandalini et al., 2000; Saavedra et al., 1994; Shornikova, 1997).

Although no manufactured probiotic pharmaceutical product has been specifically tested on childbearing women, there are no reports of harm. As such, probiotic products are freely sold in supermarkets. Lack of research focus in the area of childbearing women means there is no direct evidence-based information from which maternity care providers can give direct advice about probiotic consumption. Beneficial effects for childbearing women can at present only be inferred from studies conducted on the non pregnant adult population.

Immune system

Probiotics are believed to boost immune function, inhibit growth of harmful bacteria and increase resistance to some infections and disease-causing bacteria. Some evidence supports that human immune function may be facilitated by growing the number of IgA populating plasma cells, T lymphocytes, natural killer cells and improving phagocytosis in the individual (Reid et al., 2003; Ouwehand, 2002). As such, it may be advantageous to take probiotics in conjunction with antibiotics, since probiotic friendly bacteria facilitate the immune system to defend the body from pathogenic invaders. A study conducted in Pennsylvania School of Medicine (2010) found that Antibiotic Associated diarrhea (AAD) and Clostridium Difficile Infection (CDI) are common side-effects from taking broad-spectrum antibiotic therapy. In a prospective study, AAD was observed in 4.9% of patients who took long standing antibiotic medication, with 50% of participants proving positive for Clostridium Difficile toxin B (Wistrom, 2001). Since incidence of CDI is on the increase (McDonald, 2006), this emphasizes a requirement for preventative strategies to reduce rates of infection. Probiotics have been shown to reduce AAD and CDI through facilitating regeneration of intestinal microbiota, when antibiotic treatment is administered simultaneously (Hickson et al., 2007; McFarland, 2006, 2009). Evidence promotes that introducing healthy bacteria into the GI tract helps maintain immune system activity, which in sequence assists the human body to respond more rapidly to new infections. Consequently, promoting probiotic intake may be more effective than prescribing antibiotics that decrease effectiveness of the immune system by eradicating communal friendly GI tract bacteria.

Probiotics that protect humans against infection (Hickson et al., 2007; McFarland, 2006, 2009) and enhance the immune system are of particular interest to midwives and obstetricians. Pregnancy is a time when childbearing women and the developing foetus require protection from teratogenic effects of pathogenic organisms that cause infection. The term teratogenic in this context means substances or agents that interfere with normal embryonic development. Acknowledging perceived benefits of probiotics at preventing infection, invites interest in propagating studies that aim to improve obstetric and neonatal outcomes in this area of research. Probiotics do not appear to have teratogenic effects, whilst many pharmaceutical products do. For example, thalidomide is an anti-emetic known to create serious foetal defects. Historically thalidomide was prescribed during 1957–1961 and was withdrawn because it was identified to specifically cause foetal limb deformities. When advising pregnant women about treatments that alleviate complications, such as GI upsets, health professionals must be vigilant and careful about the recommendations they make. According to the literature, probiotics appear to be highly effective at helping prevent infection and work towards reducing GI tract discomfort. RCTs that measure effects of taking probiotics and their benefits in terms of reducing morning sickness, heartburn, constipation and reducing GI tract infections during pregnancy would create greater insights into the benefits for childbearing women and neonates.

Cardiovascular system

Although unconfirmed, some studies have indicated that consumption of milk fermented with LAB produces a small reduction in blood pressure, with this effect thought to be related to ACE inhibitor peptides produced during fermentation (Sanders, 2000). In relation to developing pre-eclampsia, or in the case where a childbearing woman has a history of high blood pressure, probiotics may prove a useful natural method of reducing such complications during pregnancy. Pre-eclampsia is a hypertensive condition unique to pregnancy that is associated with high blood pressure, oedema and significant amounts of protein in the urine. Complications of pre-eclampsia include damage to the maternal endothelium, kidneys and liver, with release of vasoconstrictive factors that are secondary to original damage. Pre-eclampsia is one of the most common dangerous pregnancy complications that effects both mother and foetus adversely (Lyall and Belfort, 2007), with an RCT to measure effects on blood pressure from taking probiotics in childbearing women possibly set to produce interesting results.

What is more, LAB has been shown to lower cholesterol levels through dismantling bile in the GI system and reducing re-absorption into the circulatory system (Sanders, 2000). A meta-analysis by Agerholm-Larsen et al. (2002) involved 5 double blind RCTs that focused upon effects of yoghurt containing probiotic strains on serum cholesterol levels over a 2–8 week period, which resulted in an alteration of 8.5 mg/dL (0.22 mmol/L) (4% decrease) in blood cholesterol and a decrease of 7.7 mg/dL (0.2 mmol/L) (5% decrease) in LDL concentration. Although none of this research focused specifically on childbearing women the results are still of interest to maternity care experts.

Genito Urinary (GU) Tract

Probiotics are considered to supercede harmful organisms with their presence in live yoghurt used to treat vaginitis. Bacterial vaginosis is a condition in which lactobacilli are dislodged from the vagina by inflammation-causing pathogens (Cauci, 2003) thought by some to precurse preterm labour (Jacobsson, 2002).

The neonate

Research supports that consuming a high quality diet during pregnancy enhances the likelihood of delivering a healthy infant that is less inclined to develop heart disease and diabetes in later life (Cauci et al., 2003). Researchers have studied probiotics to identify whether they reduce risk of premature birth and risks of the childbearing woman delivering a Low Birth Weight (LBW) infant. A LBW infant is a newborn that weighs less than is 2,500 grams regardless of gestational age. Findings from studies are mixed, with one cause of premature labour thought to be infection that stimulates an imbalance of communal microorganisms and prevents pathogens from multiplying, which is what occurs in vaginal thrush.

Lactobacillus reuteri have shown to be effective at treating infant colic. Savino et al. (2010) conducted a double-blind placebo-controlled RCT that involved exclusively breast-fed and colicky infants (n = 50) and found a significant decrease in daily crying time when adminstered *Lactobacillus reuteri* compared to a placebo group. A significant increase in *Lactobacilli* colonization, a decrease in faecal *Escherichia coli* and ammonia was also identified. Precisely how *Lactobacillus reuteri* alleviates symptoms of colic remains unclear, with infants becoming ill less often, visiting the doctor less frequently, and reduced absenteeism from child care compared with a placebo group (Weizman et al., 2005).

In addition, more research is required to ascertain whether premature labour can be prevented through probiotic use. RCT's have shown that probiotics reduce dental caries in children (Näse et al., 2001) and decrease incidence of acquiring Respiratory Tract Infections (RTI) (Hatakka et al., 2001), with this of particular interest to premature neonates who have a predisposition to developing RTI's. Tissier (1900) discovered that breast milk contains natural *prebiotics* that facilitate growth of advantageous bacteria in the GI tract. He isolated Bifidobacterium found amongst GI flora of breast fed babies and identified clinical benefits in terms of treating diarrhea. Such protection is one of the long recognized benefits about which to inform childbearing women when advising about benefits of breastfeeding.

Skin conditions

Probiotics have been studied to identify whether they reduce the incidence of developing allergic conditions such as eczema in the newborn (Vanderhoof, 2008). *L. rhamnosus GG* and *B. lactis BB12* has been used to treat atopic dermatitis, which occurs in around 15% of neonates, with figures halved when women took oral probiotics prenatally (Kalliomaki et al., 2001; Kankaanpaa, 2002). Again, neonatal skin protection afforded by probiotics is important information to impart to childbearing women and an area that merits further research attention.

Discussion

Media messages espouse benefits of consuming probiotics. In the main it is still speculative how effective, in what dosage and packaging and what outcomes may be effected by probiotics use. Also, amounts of probiotic content in consumable foods differ considerably. So what advice do midwives, general practitioners, health visitors, obstetricians and paediatric nurses give to childbearing women about probiotic use? Quite clearly, more studies are required to explore relationships between probiotics, childbearing women and neonatal health to enhance understanding of interactions with physical, psychological and social reproductive processes. What we do know is that probiotics do not cause harm. For maternity health care professionals there are a whole host of unanswered research questions. For example:

- What probiotic food products are safe to consume during pregnancy and in what quantity?
- What is the evidence-base about preventing and treating specified complications during pregnancy with probiotics?
- What are the effects of taking probiotics upon sickness, heartburn, constipation and incidence of GI tract infections during pregnancy?

Taking probiotics whilst pregnant has a positive safety record (Reid, 2002), which is encouraging, since pregnancy is a time to consider carefully what one consumes. No group of women has as many minor disorders as childbearing women, with the vast array of hormones and growth patterns of pregnancy often causing heartburn, diarrhoea, constipation and cramping (Jones, 1999).

Research about probiotics and childbearing and the effects on the neonate is still in its infancy, with rigorous RCTs required to evidence benefits during pregnancy and for newborns. To date research has shown most about the role of probiotics in promoting healthy GI tract functioning (Guandalini et al., 2000; Mach, 2006; Ouwehand, 2002; Reid et al., 2003; Saavedra et al., 1994; Shornikova, 1997; Yan and Polk, 2006). *Lactobacillus reuteri* has been tested for host tolerance in healthy adults (Wolf et al., 1995), the young (Ruiz-Palaccious et al., 1992) and those who are immunosuppressed (Wolf et al., 1998), with no undesirable medical side effects observed on giving the highest prescription of 10^{10} CFUs per day and no significant differences in blood count, urinalysis, metabolism and liver function tests between participants taking *Lactobacillus reuteri* or a placebo. What is clear is that there is a lack of research focus and minimal evidence-base from which to advise childbearing women in relation to probiotic consumption. Data can only be inferred from studies conducted on the non-pregnant adult population. To gain the advantage of probiotic consumption, childbearing woman are not required to take oral probiotic tablets or capsules. Instead benefits may be gained from eating natural foodstuffs that are high in probiotic content, such as yoghurts and yoghurt drinks (see Table 1). Advice on how to ingest the right probiotics through daily recipe planning is one approach, along with providing information about naturally occurring probiotic compounds and how to gain benefits through supplementation.

Conclusion

The most researched area in probiotic study relates to promoting healthy GI tract function (Bakken et al., 2011; Borody et al., 2011; Guandalini et al., 2000; Hickson et al., 2007; McFarland, 2006, 2009; Shornikova, 1997; Mach, 2006; Saavedra et al., 1994; Yan and Polk, 2006). Of greater significance, perhaps is the potential of using probiotics to boost the immune system of both mother and newborn. As more rigorous RCTs are conducted in relation to advantages of childbearing women taking probiotics, midwives and obstetricians will grow confident to encourage their intake. In the future, and post further research, potentially probiotics may be added to multivitamin supplements routinely prescribed during pregnancy. Childbearing women taking probiotics may reap rewards in terms of the immune system and allergy prevention. At a global level, benefits from taking probiotics are an ongoing issue for researchers. Given how merciless disorders of pregnancy can be, adding beneficial bacteria in the form of probiotics to the woman's immune system may be a cheap and effortless attempt to alleviate unpleasant experiences. It is important for maternity care professionals to appreciate that where the childbearing woman has a complicated pregnancy, malady, or is taking treatments for a diagnosed condition, they should seek approval for taking probiotics from their doctor.

References

Abrahamsson T, Jakobsson T, Sinkiewicz G, Fredriksson M and Björkstén B (2005) Intestinal microbiota in infants supplemented with the probiotic bacterium *Lactobacillus reuteri*. Journal of Pediatric Gastroenterol Nutrition 40: 692.

Açikgöz ZC, Gamberzade S, Göçer S and Ceylan P (2005) Fatih Universitesi Tip Fakültesi, Mikrobiyoloji ve Klinik Mikrobiyoloji—Inhibitor effect of vaginal lactobacilli on group B streptococci. Mikrobiyol Bul 39: 17–23.

Agerholm-Larsen L, Bell ML, Grunwald GK and Astrup A (2002) The effect of a probiotic milk product on plasma cholesterol: a meta-analysis of short term intervention studies. European Journal of Clinical Nutrition 54: 856–860.

Anukam KC, Osazuwa EO and Reid G (2005) Improved appetite of pregnant rats and increased birth weight of newborns following feeding with probiotic *Lactobacillus rhamnosus* GR-1 and *L. fermentum* RC-14. Journal of Applied Research 5: 46–52.

Bakken JS, Borody TJ, Brandt LJ, Brill JV, Demarco DC, Franzos MA, Kelly C, Khoruts A, Louie T, Martinelli LP, Moore TA, Russell G and Surawicz C (2011) Treating Clostridium *difficile* infection with fecal microbiota transplantation. Clinical Gastroenterology and Hepatology 9: 1044–1049.

Borody TJ and Campbell J (2011) Fecal microbiota transplantation: current status and future directions. Expert Review of Gastroenterology and Hepatology 5: 653–655.

Boyle RJ, Bath-Hextall FJ, Leonardi-Bee J, Murrell DF and Tang ML (2009) Probiotics for the treatment of eczema: a systematic review. Clinical & Experimental Allergy 39: 1117–27.

Buts JP, Bernasconi P, Vaerman JP and Dive C (1990) Stimulation of secretory IgA and secretory component of immunoglobulins in small intestine of rats treated with *Saccharomyces boulardii*. Digestive Diseases and Science 35: 251–6.

Canaani RB, Cirillo P, Terrin G, Cesarano L, Spagnuolo MI, De Vincenzo A, Albano F, Passariello A, De Marco G, Manguso F and Guarino A (2007) Probiotics for treatment of accute diarrhoea in children: RCT of 5 different preparations. British Medical Journal 335: 340.

Castagliuolo I, Riegler MF, Valenick L, LaMont JT and Pothoulakis C (1999) *Saccharomyces boulardii* protease inhibits the effects of Clostridium difficile toxins A and B in colonic mucosa. Infection and Immunity 67: 302–7.

Cauci S, Guaschino S, De Aloysio D, Driussi S, De Santo D and Penacchioni P (2003) Interrelationships of interleukin-8 with interleukin-1beta and neutrophils in vaginal fluid of healthy and bacterial vaginosis positive women. Molecular Human Reproduction 9: 53–58.

Challa SK (2012) Probiotics for dummies. Wiley, London.

Cleusix V, Lacroix C, Vollenweider S and Le Blay G (2008) Glycerol induces reuterin production and decreases *Escherichia coli* population in an *in vitro* model of colonic fermentation with immobilized human feces. FEMS Microbiol Ecol 63: 56–64.

Dugoua J, Machado M, Zhu X, Chen X, Koren G and Einarson TR (2009) Probiotic safety in pregnancy: a systematic review and meta-analysis of randomized controlled trials of lactobacillus, bifidobacterium, and saccharomyces. Journal of Obstetrics and Gynaecology Canada 31(6): 542–552.

Gedek BR (1999) Adherence of *Escherichia coli* serogroup O 157 and the Salmonella typhimurium mutant DT 104 to the surface of *Saccharomyces boulardii*. Mycoses 42: 261–4.

Guandalini S, Pensabene L, Zikri MA, Dias JA, Casali LG, Hoekstra H, Kolacek S, Massar K, Micetic-Turk D, Papadopoulou A, de Sousa JS, Sandhu B, Szajewska H and Weizman Z (2000) *Lactobacillus GG* administered in oral rehydration solution to children with acute diarrhea: a multicenter European trial. Journal of Pediatric Gastroenetrol Nutrition 30: 54–60.

Hamilton-Miller JM, Gibson GR and Bruck W (2003) Some insights into the derivation and early uses of the word probiotic. British Journal of Nutrition 845.

Hatakka K, Savilahti E, Pönkä A, Meurman JH, Poussa T, Näse L, Saxelin M and Korpela R (2001) Effects of long term consumption of probiotic milk on infections in children attending day care centres: double blind randomised trial. British Medical Journal 322: 1327.

Havenaar R and Huis In't Veld JMJ (1992) Probiotics: a general view. *In*: Lactic Acid Bacteria in Health and Disease (Vol. 1). Elsevier Applied Science Publishers.

Hickson M, D'Souza AL, Muthu N, Rogers TR, Want S, Rajkumar C and Bulpitt CJ (2007) Use of probiotic Lactobacillus preparation to prevent diarrhoea associated with antibiotics: randomised double blind placebo controlled trial. British Medical Journal 335: 80.

Hojsak I, Snovak N, Abdović S, Szajewska H, Mišak Z and Kolaček S (2009) *Lactobacillus GG* in the prevention of gastrointestinal and respiratory tract infections in children who attend day care centers: A randomized, double-blind, placebo-controlled trial. Clinical Nutrition 29: 312–6.

Imase K, Tanaka A, Tokunaga K, Sugano H, Ishida H and Takahashi S (2007) *Lactobacillus reuteri* tablets suppress *Helicobacter pylori* infection: a double-blind randomised placebo-controlled cross-over clinical study. Kansenshōgaku Zasshi 81: 387–93.

Jacobsson B, Pernevi P, Chidekel L and Platz-Christensen J (2002) Bacterial vaginosis in early pregnancy may predispose for preterm birth and postpartum endometritis. Acta Obstetricia et Gynecologica Scandinavica 81: 1006–1010.

Jones K (1999) Relief of heartburn and constipation during pregnancy. British Journal of Midwifery 7: 228–230.

Kalliomaki M, Salminen S, Arvilommi H, Kero P, Koskinen P and Isolauri E (2001) Probiotics in primary prevention of atopic disease: a randomised placebo-controlled trial. Lancet 357: 1076–1079.

Kalliomäki M, Salminen S, Poussa T and Isolauri E (2007) Probiotics during the first 7 years of life: a cumulative risk reduction of eczema in a randomized, placebo-controlled trial. Journal of Allergy and Clinical Immunology 119: 1019–21.

Kandler O, Stetter K and Kohl R (1980) *Lactobacillus reuteri* sp. nov. a new species of heterofermentative lactobacilli. Zbl Bakt Hyg Abt Orig C1: 264–9.

Kankaanpaa PE, Yang B, Kallio HP, Isolauri E and Salminen SJ (2002) Influence of probiotic supplemented infant formula on composition of plasma lipids in atopic infants. Journal of Nutritional Biochemistry 13(6): 364–369.

Krasse P, Carlsson B, Dahl C, Paulsson A, Nilsson A and Sinkiewicz G (2006) Decreased gum bleeding and reduced gingivitis by the probiotic *Lactobacillus reuteri*. Swedish Dental Journal 30: 55–60.

Lyall F and Belfort M (2007) Pre-eclampsia: Etiology and Clinical Practice. Cambridge University Press.

Mach T (2006) Clinical usefulness of probiotics in inflammatory bowel diseases. Journal of Physiology and Pharmacology 57: 23–33.

Manley KJ, Fraenkel MB, Mayall BC and Power DA (2007) Probiotic treatment of vancomycin-resistant enterococci: a randomised controlled trial. Medical Journal of Australia 186: 454–7.

McDonald LC, Owings M and Jernigan DB (2006) Clostridium difficile infection in patients discharged from US short-stay hospitals 1996–2003. Emergency Infectious Diseases 12: 409–415.

McFarland LV (2006) Meta-analysis of probiotics for the prevention of antibiotic associated diarrhea and the treatment of Clostridium difficile disease. American Journal of Gastroenterology 101: 812–822.

McFarland LV (2009) Evidence-based review of probiotics for antibiotic associated diarrhea and Clostridium difficile infections. Anaerobe 15: 274–280.

Näse L, Hatakka K and Savilahti E (2001) Effect of long-term consumption of a probiotic bacterium, *Lactobacillus rhamnosus* GG, in milk on dental caries and caries risk in children. Caries Research 35(6): 412–20.

Nikawa H, Makihira S and Fukushima H (2004) *Lactobacillus reuteri* in bovine milk fermented decreases the oral carriage of mutans streptococci. International Journal of Food Microbiology 95: 219–23.

Osborn DA and Sinn JK (2007) Probiotics in infants for prevention of allergic disease and food hypersensitivity. Cochrane Database Syst. Rev. CD006475.

Österlund P, Ruotsalainen T, Korpela R, Saxelin M, Ollus A, Valta P, Kouri M, Elomaa I and Joensuu H (2007) Lactobacillus supplementation for diarrhoea related to chemotherapy of colorectal cancer: a randomised study 97: 1028–34.

Ouwehand AC, Salminen S and Isolauri E (2002) Probiotics: an overview of beneficial effetcs. Antonie Van Leeuwenhoek 82: 279–89.

Reid G, Beuerman D, Heinemann C and Bruce AW (2001) Probiotic *Lactobacillus* dose required to restore and maintain a normal vaginal flora. FEMS Immunology and Medical Microbiology 32: 37–41.

Reid G (2002) Safety of *Lactobacillus* strains as probiotic agents. Clinical Infectious Diseases 35: 349–350.

Reid G, Hammond JA and Bruce AW (2003) Effect of lactobacilli oral supplement on the vaginal microflora of antibiotic treated patients: randomized, placebo-controlled study. Nutraceut Food 8: 145–148.

Reid G, Jass J, Sebulsky MT and McCormick JK (2003) Potential uses of probiotics in clinical practice. Clinical Microbiology Review 16(4): 658–72.

Reid G, Burton J, Hammond JA and Bruce AW (2004) Nucleic acid based diagnosis of bacterial vaginosis and improved management using probiotic lactobacilli. Journal of Medicinal Food 7: 223–228.

Reid G (2008) Probiotic Lactobacilli for urogenital health in women. Journal of Clinical Gastroenterology 42: 234–6.

Roberfroid MB (2007) Prebiotics: the concept revisited. The Journal of Nutrition 137: 830–837.

Ruiz-Palacios G, Tuz F, Arteaga F, Guerrero ML, Dohnalek M and Hilty M (1992) Tolerance and fecal colonization with *Lactobacillus reuteri* in children fed a beverage with a mixture of *Lactobacillus* spp. Pediatric Research 39: 1090.

Saavedra JM, Bauman NA, Oung I, Perman JA and Yolken RH (1994) Feeding of *Bifidobacterium bifidum* and *Streptococcus thermophilus* to infants in hospital for prevention of diarrhoea and shedding of rotavirus. Lancet 344: 1046–1049.

Saint-Marc T, Blehaut H, Musial C and Touraine J (1995) AIDS related diarrhea: a double-blind trial of *Saccharomyces boulardii*. Sem Hôsp Paris 71: 735–41.

Sanders ME (2000) Considerations for use of probiotic bacteria to modulate human health. The Journal of Nutrition 130: 384–390.

Sanders ME (2003) Probiotics: considerations for human health. Nutrition Review 61: 91–99.

Savino F, Cordisco L, Tarasco V, Palumeri E, Calabrese R, Oggero R, Roos S and Matteuzzi D (2010) *Lactobacillus reuteri* DSM 17938 in infantile colic: A randomized, double-blind, placebo-controlled trial. Pediatrics 126: e526–e533.

Schrezenmeir J and de Vrese M (2001) Probiotics, prebiotics, and synbiotics—approaching a definition. American Journal of Clinical Nutrition 73: 361–364.

Shornikova AV, Casas IA, Isolauri E, Mykkanen H and Vesikari T (1997) *Lactobacillus reuteri* as a therapeutic agent in acute diarrhea in young children. Journal of Pediatric Gastroenterology and Nutrition 24: 399–404.

Sinkiewicz G and Nordström EA (2005) Occurrence of *Lactobacillus reuteri*, lactobacilli and bifidobacteria in human breast milk. Pediatric Research 58(2): 415.

Tissier H (1900) Recherchers sur la flora intestinale normale et pathologique du nourisson. Thesis, University of Paris, Paris, France.

Tubelius P, Stan V and Zachrisson A (2005) Increasing work-place healthiness with the probiotic *Lactobacillus reuteri*: a randomised, double-blind placebo-controlled study. Environmental Health 4: 25.

University of Pennsylvania School of Medicine (2010) Good bacteria keeps the immune system primed to fight future infections. Science Daily. Available at: http://www.sciencedaily.com/releases/2010/01/100127095945.htm. Accessed on 3rd September 2012.

Vanderhoof JA (2008) Probiotics in allergy management. Journal of Pediatric Gastroenterology and Nutrition 47: 38–40.

Weizman Z, Asli G and Alsheikh A (2005) Effect of a probiotic infant formula on infections in child care centers: comparison of two probiotic agents. Pediatrics 115: 5–9.

Wiström J, Norrby SR, Myhre EB, Eriksson S, Granstorm G, Englund G, Nord CE and Svenungsson B (2001) Frequency of antibiotic-associated diarrhoea in 2462 antibiotic-treated hospitalized patients: a prospective study. Journal of Antimicrobial Chemotherapy 47(1): 43–50.

Wolf BW, Garleb KA, Ataya DG and Casas IA (1995) Safety and tolerance of *Lactobacillus reuteri* in healthy adult male subjects. Microbial Ecology in Health and Disease 8(2): 41–50.

Wolf BW, Wheeler KB, Ataya DG and Garleb KA (1998) Safety and tolerance of *Lactobacillus reuteri* supplementation to a population infected with the human immunodeficiency virus. Food and Chemical Toxicology 36: 1085–94.

World Health Organisation (WHO) (2001) Expert consultation on evaluation of health and nutritional properties of probiotics in food including powder milk with live Lactic Acid Bacteria. Food and Agricultural Organisation of the United Nations. Available at: http://www.who.int/foodsafety/publications/fs_management/en/probiotics.pdf. Accessed 2nd Sptember 2012.

Yan F and Polk DB (2006) Probiotics as functional food in the treatment of diarrhea. Current Opinion in Clinical Nutrition and Metabolic Care 9: 717–21.

CHAPTER 6

Mechanisms of Action of Probiotics in Psychopathology

Moira S Lewitt

INTRODUCTION

This chapter will focus on the actions of probiotics, live microorganisms that, when administered in adequate amounts to humans and animals, confer a health benefit (Joint FAO/WHO Expert Consultation, 2001). Prebiotics, dietary substances that favour beneficial bacteria in the gut microbiome, and synbiotics, containing a mixture of probiotics and prebiotics, are distinct areas that will not be addressed in this review. It should be emphasised that these working definitions are functional ones. While increasing numbers of research reports demonstrate the effect of probiotics on specific human diseases, few address the underlying mechanisms of action. Since the range of activity that is reported is wide, it is also likely that the underlying mechanisms are diverse. Although the specificity of action, and not the source of the organism, is considered most important (Joint FAO/WHO Expert Consultation, 2001), evidence is now emerging that some actions may prove to be species- and even strain-specific.

It is now well recognised that the organisms of the gastrointestinal tract make important contributions to health and disease, including mood and cognition, and psychopathology. In this review I will first summarise our current understanding of how the gut microbiome contributes generally to health and well-being, and then focus on the pathways connecting the microbiome to CNS function: the microbiome-gut–brain axis. The potential molecular mechanisms, particularly those that support a role for probiotics in the management of psychopathology, will then be reviewed and recommendations made for future research in this area.

University of the West of Scotland, Paisley Campus, Paisley, Scotland, PA1 2BE.
Email: Moira.Lewitt@uws.ac.uk

Contribution of the Microbiome to Human Health and Well-being

In health, the human gastrointestinal tract is host to around 10^{14} bacteria, known as the gut microbiota and representing a bacterial genome, or microbiome, that outnumbers the number of human genes by two orders of magnitude. This diversity is the result of co-evolutionary selection pressures between the microbiota and host, and also between gut microbial communities (Ley et al., 2006). On the whole, this is a mutually beneficial relationship that is believed to contribute to human health by preventing infectious, inflammatory and allergic diseases. It is now emerging that the gut microbiota also contributes to human nutrition, and to brain development and behaviour. Products of the gut microbiota are also involved in the biotransformation of potential carcinogens (Guarner and Malagelada, 2003). Disturbance in the gut microbiota, interacting with other environmental factors and the host genotype, may therefore contribute to a range of diseases, including psychopathology.

Contribution to Digestion and Nutrition

It is well established that the gut microbiota plays an important role within the gastrointestinal tract (Macpherson and Harris, 2004; Mai and Draganov, 2009). It is essential for normal motility and in maintenance of a normal gastrointestinal barrier. The latter involves induction of epithelial cell proliferation through recognition of molecules, known as pathogen-associated molecular patterns (PAMPs), by toll-like receptors (TLRs) on the epithelial cell surface (Rakoff-Nahoum et al., 2004). The gastrointestinal barrier is also maintained against invasion by pathogenic bacteria, through competition for attachment sites and nutrition at the epithelial brush border. In addition, the microbiota releases a variety of antimicrobial peptides, including α-defensins.

Research studies using rodents bred in a germ-free environment demonstrate the role of the gut biota in host development and health. Germ free animals require more calories to maintain their body weight compared to controls (Sumi et al., 1977). The metabolic activities of the microbiota provide the host with some nutrients indirectly, by modulating absorption, as well as directly, for example by providing phylloquinone (vitamin K1) and short chain fatty acids through the metabolism of dietary fibre. Recognition that gut microbiota are involved in nutrient processing has led to speculation that individuals at risk of obesity have a microbiome that contributes greater nutrition to the host (Turnbaugh et al., 2006). It is also hypothesised that part of the epigenetic effect of nutrition on gene expression might be through the development and function of the gut microbiota, and this may be one of the factors responsible for the increased incidence of obesity and type 2 diabetes (Canani et al., 2011).

Development of Immune Tolerance

Studies in germ-free mice clearly show that commensal gut organisms have a key role in lymphoid tissue development, and the development of a competent local and systemic immune system (Macpherson and Harris, 2004). Organisms that cross the gastrointestinal barrier, although destroyed by macrophages, can survive, and have activity in dendritic cells associated with the gut mucosa. The gut microbiota are required for the expression of TLRs on a variety of immune cells, resulting in IgA secretion, cytokine production and T cell activation (Ulevitch, 1999; Wells et al., 2011). Commensal flora are required for a fully functional regulatory T cell population and production of the anti-inflammatory cytokine interleukin-10 (□acpherson and Harris, 2004; Ostman et al., 2006). A disturbance of this controlled inflammatory response, will lead to pathological inflammation and disease. Reduced local tolerance due to changes in the gut microbiota, for example, is likely to contribute to inflammatory bowel disease.

Contribution to CNS Development and Function

The perinatal period is a time during which the gut is rapidly populated by microorganisms. It is also an important time for brain development. Studies in germ-free mice suggest that the gut microbiota is important in this process and may have an impact on host behaviour in adult life (Diaz Heijtz et al., 2011). This critical developmental window is also essential in the development of an appropriate stress response. Germ-free mice have an exaggerated corticosterone and ACTH response to restraint stress, that is reversed by microbial colonisation (Sudo et al., 2004).

The gut microbiota synthesises a vast array of neurotransmitters, including -aminobutyric acid (GABA), melatonin and tryptophan, which may mediate the effect of neuronal development and plasticity. Epigenetic mechanisms may also have a role: it has been demonstrated that there are long lasting epigenetic effects on neural development and mature neurones and therefore on complex behaviour (Tsankova et al., 2007). In mice, offspring of high nurturing mothers have less anxious behaviours, attenuated corticosterone responses to stress and increased expression of an alternatively spliced variant of the glucocorticoid receptor, that is modified by central infusion of a histone deacetylase inhibitor (Weaver et al., 2004). The role of the gut microbiota in these responses is yet to be explored.

The Microbiome-Gut–Brain Axis

In the 1930s Stokes and Pillsbury proposed the use of Lactobacillus acidophilus for the treatment of acne vulgaris, on the basis of a unifying theory for the disease: the gut–brain-skin axis (Bowe and Logan, 2011). Their central hypothesis, illustrated in Figure 1, was that acne is frequently associated with psychopathology, particularly anxiety and depression, and this was causally related to altered GI tract function, and altered microbial flora, which then induced local and systemic inflammation. Clinical studies continue to support the theory by demonstrating that probiotics have a role in the treatment of simple acne (Bowe and Logan, 2011).

The idea that there is a connection between "gut health" and brain function is therefore not new. Nevertheless, potential mechanisms underlying this connection are only now emerging, and we are still a long way from understanding its complexity. The effect of gut on brain and the effect of stress on the gut microbiota and normal gastrointestinal function are the subject of recent reviews (Collins and Bercik, 2009; Konturek et al., 2011; Dinan and Cryan, 2012). The "forgotten

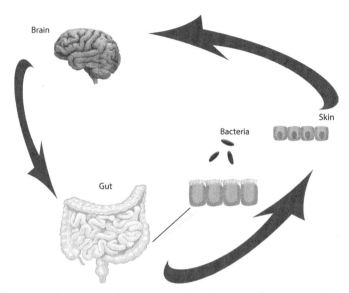

Figure 1 The Gut–Brain-Skin connection was proposed by Stokes and Pillsbury as a unifying mechanism underlying the overlap between acne, anxiety and depression (see Bowe and Logan, 2011). Altered normal intestinal microflora and increased intestinal permeability were proposed to result in systemic inflammation.

organ", the microbiome, is now well established as a participant in the gut–brain axis. Summarised in Figure 2, this axis comprises bidirectional pathways involving immune, neural and endocrine signals.

The most dramatic evidence for a link between the gut microbiome and brain is the altered cognitive function that accompanies severe liver disease. Neurotoxins derived from the gut microbiota play a pathological role in hepatic encephalopathy and oral non-absorbable antibiotics are now standard treatment (Rothenberg and Keeffe, 2005). Systemic infections can also have central effects that relate to the action of pro-inflammatory mediators (Dantzer et al., 2008), ranging from "sickness behaviour" that may be appropriately adaptive, so that individuals cope better with illness, through to clinical depression. Conversely, depression and anxiety, as primary disorders, are associated with changes in pro-inflammatory cytokines that contribute to changes in neuroendocrine pathways and neurotransmitters (Anisman and Merali, 2003; Alesci et al., 2005). There are a number of theories as to how pro-inflammatory cytokines from the periphery, such TNF-alpha, interleukin-1beta and interleukin-6, cross the blood-brain barrier or whether the primary effect is at the cerebral vascular endothelium (Takeshita and Ransohoff, 2012). Peripherally produced cytokines may stimulate a cascade of central *de novo* cytokine synthesis centrally, mainly by glial cells, which contribute to the sickness response, including pain facilitation (Watkins and Maier, 2005).

Although it has long been recognised that major disturbances in gut flora can affect central nervous system function, it is only now emerging that "normal" gut microbiota might have a role in mood and psychopathology (Forsythe et al., 2010). Both endocrine and neural pathways are involved in signalling gut immune responses to brain. The neural pathways involved in the microbiome-gut–brain axis include the sympathetic and parasympathetic autonomic nervous system and the local enteric nervous system. The myenteric and submucous plexuses that make up the enteric nervous system comprise sympathetic and parasympathetic efferent, as well as vagal and lower dorsal root ganglia afferent fibres. The molecular patterns of bacterial and viral components are recognised by TLRs that are also expressed neurons that make up the enteric nervous system (Rumio et al., 2006; Rolls et al., 2007; Barajon et al., 2009). The neuroimmune pathways stimulated by the gut microbiota also involve production by dendritic cells of anti-inflammatory cytokines, including interleukin-10 and the suppression of pro-inflammatory cytokine production. Locally produced cytokines directly activate vagus nerve afferents that terminate in the nucleus tractus solitarius, which is known to be involved in the sickness response. There is also indirect activation through involvement of paraganglia (Goehler et al., 1999).

The pathways are bidirectional—the mucosal response to bacterial antigens is modified by neural and endocrine signals from the brain. Host stress induces changes in the microbial environment, including changes in gastrointestinal motility, gastric acid production, and intestinal permeability and mucoid production. Neural and endocrine pathways, in turn, can alter the immune response (Watkins and Maier, 2005). Macrophages, for example, respond to glucocorticoids, catecholamines and acetylcholine. Furthermore stress-related signalling molecules that reach the gut lumen, including serotonin, may have a direct impact on the microbiota (Rhee et al.,

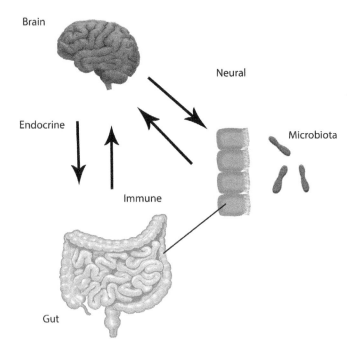

Figure 2 The Microbiome-Gut–Brain axis comprises immune, neural and endocrine pathways that are bidirectional.

2009; Grenham et al., 2011). Noradrenaline from the host, for example, has been shown to increase the virulence of pathogenic bacteria (Cogan et al., 2007).

Potential Mechanisms of Probiotic Action in Psychopathology

Metchnikoff proposed that consumption of viable microbes might improve health by replacing harmful microbes by useful ones (Metchnikoff, 1907). Most probiotics currently in use are also part of the normal gut flora. Lactobacilli contribute to the small intestinal microbiota, and Bifidobacteria to the colon. It is believed that the primary mechanisms of action of probiotics are to contribute to, and/or modify, the functions of the gut microbiota. Parental routes of administration however have also been proposed (Sheil et al., 2004, 53: 694).

The effect probiotics on the entire microbiome-gut–brain axis is not yet defined. This section therefore reviews the potential mechanisms involving the known immune, neural and endocrine pathways of the gut–brain axis. These are illustrated in Figure 3.

Actions on the microbiome-gut–brain axis may be direct or indirect. Altering the resident gut microbiota, for example by inhibiting bacterial interaction/adhesion to epithelial cells, competing for nutrients or secreting bactericidal proteins, may indirectly alter the function of this axis. Several cell-surface associated adhesion proteins have been identified in Lactobacillus acidophilus (Buck et al., 2005).

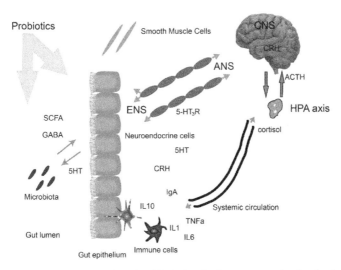

Figure 3 Potential mechanisms of action of probiotics involve immune, neural and endocrine signalling pathways. Probiotics may influence the enteric nervous system (ENS) and central nervous system (CNS) via pathways that involve the autonomic nervous system (ANS) as well as immune and neuroendocrine signalling. The putative molecular basis is described in the text and includes involvement of serotonin (5HT) and it receptor (5-HT$_3$R), γ-aminobutyric acid (GABA), short-chain fatty acids (SCFA), immunoglobulin A (IgA), anti-inflammatory cytokine interleukin 10 (IL10), pro-inflammatory cytokines (IL1, IL6 and tumour necrosis factor-α (TNFα)) and the components of the hypothalamic-pituitary-adrenal (HPA) axis (corticotrophin releasing hormone (CRH), adrenocorticotrophic hormone (ACTH) and cortisol).

The host microbiota may in turn affect probiotic action. It is known that molecules (e.g., noradrenaline, dynorphins, cytokines) produced by the host can affect the pathogenicity of gut microorganisms. It is also speculated that these, and other molecules (e.g., serotonin, corticotrophin releasing hormone (CRH)), secreted by enterochromaffin, nerve and immune cells, may modify probiotics actions.

Immune Pathways

Since the gut microbiota has a crucial role in the development of innate and adaptive immune responses, the potential of probiotics to stimulate immunity is of central interest. Administration of lactobacillus species in animals and man have been shown to act on dendritic cells to induce production of regulatory T cells and cytokine synthesis, particularly interleukin-10 (reviews by (Boirivant and Strober, 2007; Forsythe et al., 2010)). Interleukin-10 is both anti-inflammatory, and nociceptive (Duncker et al., 2008) and probiotics may potentially influence mood by either of these pathways. It is not known whether these actions of probiotics require whole organisms or their components. Live Lactobacillus reuteri is required to inhibit TNF-alpha-induced interleukin-8 in a mouse model of colitis (Ma et al., 2004). This effect was not mimicked by the use of cellular lysates or supernatants of culture medium. Others studies however have shown that nonviable bacteria, bacterial DNA components and probiotics-culture media can have beneficial molecular actions (Dotan and Rachmilewitz, 2005). DNA from probiotic bacteria, for example, has also been shown to have direct effects to ameliorate epithelial inflammatory responses (Jijon et al., 2004). The action of components of probiotics in psychopathology is yet to be elucidated.

Neural Pathways

The enteric nervous system may be involved in the action of probiotics. A number of bacterial strains have been shown to act on nuclear factor-κB-signaling pathways to increase the production of nerve growth factor (Ma et al., 2004). Oral administration of Lactobacillus species to rodents has been shown to diminish visceral pain perception, in association with altered enteric nervous system signalling and increased expression of epithelial μ-opioid and cannabinoid receptors (Verdu et al., 2006; Forsythe et al., 2010). These studies also demonstrated an impact on somatic pain sensitivity by mechanisms that are yet to be elucidated.

It is speculated that short chain fatty acids (e.g., butyrate and propionic acid) the products of anaerobic fermentation by the gut microbiota, may be involved in neural development and function, including behaviour. While it can be speculated that probiotics act in this way, there are as yet few studies to support this. One research group has shown that the addition of Bifidobacterium and Lactobacillus to infant formulas was associated with a reduction in the proportion of α-linoleic acid in plasma phospholipids (Kankaanpaa et al., 2002).

The gut microbiota produces a variety of neuroactive molecules, including indoles (serotonin and melatonin), catecholamines, fatty-acid derivatives (e.g., acetylcholine), histamine, gamma-aminobutyric acid and nitric oxide. It is proposed that in animals the enzymes underlying these messenger-metabolism pathways were in fact acquired in animals by a comparatively late horizontal gene transfer from bacteria (Iyer et al., 2004). The production of gamma-aminobutyric acid involves proton exchange and may serve to protect probiotics Lactobacilli in the stomach environment (Forsythe et al., 2010). A spectrum of probiotics activities may arise from production of variety of neurotransmitters. The probiotics B. Infantis 35624, for example, has been shown to induce an increase in plasma tryptophan, a precursor to serotonin (Desbonnet et al., 2008).

Exciting recent work shows that treatment of mice with Lactobacillus rhamnosus alters GABA and has an impact stress induced corticosterone and anxiety and depression-related behaviour via vagal nerve signalling (Bravo et al., 2011). To date this is the strongest evidence of a neural mechanism of action for probiotics, and also demonstrates the important connection between neural and endocrine signalling.

Endocrine Pathways

This hypothalamic-pituitary-adrenal (HPA) axis links the aetiology of depression to stressful life events in a causative manner. There is strong support for the "corticotrope hypothesis" of depression: CRH and cortisol levels are increased, and there is an impaired response during dexamethasone suppression testing (see reviews by (Forsythe et al., 2010; Massart et al., 2012)). Mice with impaired glucocorticoids receptor signalling have altered behavioural responses that are ameliorated by antidepressant treatment (□ontkowski et al., 1995). Together with pro-inflammatory cytokines, glucocorticoids alter tryptophan metabolism and lead to reduced synthesis of serotonin and increased production of kynurenin, a neurotoxic metabolite (Massart et al., 2012). Glucocorticoids appear to have important anatomical and functional effects on areas of the brain that are important to mood (e.g., hippocampus), and it appears that some of their effects on gene expression are epigenetic in nature (Massart et al., 2012). With this background, stress has been shown to change the balance and responsiveness of the gut microbiota, in an endocrine fashion (Freestone et al., 2008). Early colonisation by the gut microbiota reverses the hyperresponsiveness of the HPA axis in germ free mice (Sudo et al., 2004). Probiotic treatment of rat pups normalises the corticosterone release induced by maternal separation (Gareau et al., 2007). This effect may also turn out to have an mechanism of action that involves the vagal nerve (Bravo et al., 2011).

Future Research Directions

Psychopathology is not included in the list of health problems considered by the joint FAO/WHO expert consultation (Joint FAO/WHO Expert Consultation, 2001), and we are a long way from realising the role of probiotics in this area and their underlying mechanisms of action. This work will require a multidisciplinary approach; there are a number of areas that should be the focus of research activity.

Probiotics are a heterogeneous group. *In vitro* studies have shown that different cytokine respond to different bacterial species (Lan et al., 2005). Probiotics may also act in concert with resident microbiota. Research should focus on the development of microbiota-based screening tests in relation to relevant clinical conditions and the development of tests to match the activity of species, strains and secreted products, alone and in combination, with those clinical conditions. This will lead the way to the design of novel therapeutics for psychopathology.

Since environmental effects, such as diet, contribute to differences in the microbiome, they are therefore also likely to have an impact on probiotic's actions. The gut microbiota of the elderly is distinct from younger individuals and may contribute to disease risk (Woodmansey, 2007). Studies should therefore address variation between individuals, including the impact of ageing and community-specific effects.

Studies should focus on the importance of gut colonisation in infancy and its impact on later psychological wellbeing. This will lead to defining the place of early probiotics use to prevent psychopathology.

Summary Points

- Research suggests that the microbiome may be an effective treatment target alone or as an adjuvant, in the management of psychopathology.

- While there is evidence for the potential mechanisms of action of probiotics in psychopathology this is in area requiring extensive and rigorous research to clearly define the health benefit, to inform clinical practice and identify new molecular targets.

- Specific strains of probiotics should be studied alone, and in combination; and the impact of psychopathology on probiotic action should also be considered.

- There should be a focus on defining the mechanisms by which probiotics might contribute to the maintenance of psychological health as well as the prevention of psychopathology.

References

Alesci S, Martinez PE, Kelkar S, Ilias I, Ronsaville DS, Listwak SJ, Ayala AR, Licinio J, Gold HK, Kling □A, Chrousos GP and Gold PW (2005) □ajor depression is associated with significant diurnal elevations in plasma interleukin-6 levels, a shift of its circadian rhythm, and loss of physiological complexity in its secretion: clinical implications. The Journal of Physiology 90: 2522–30.

Anisman H and Merali Z (2003) Cytokines, stress and depressive illness: brain-immune interactions. Annals of Medicine 35: 2–11.

Barajon I, Serrao G, Arnaboldi F, Opizzi E, Ripamonti G, Balsari A and Rumio C (2009) Toll-like receptors 3, 4, and 7 are expressed in the enteric nervous system and dorsal root ganglia. Journal of Histochemistry and Cytochemistry 57: 1013–23.

Boirivant M and Strober W (2007) The mechanism of action of probiotics. Current Opinion in Gastroenterology 23: 679–92.

Bowe WP and Logan AC (2011) Acne vulgaris, probiotics and the gut–brain-skin axis—back to the future? Gut Pathogens 3: 1.

Bravo JA, Forsythe P, Chew MV, Escaravage E, Savignac HM, Dinan TG, Bienenstock J and Cryan JF (2011) Ingestion of Lactobacillus strain regulates emotional behavior and central GABA receptor expression in a mouse via the vagus nerve. Proceedings of the National Academy of Sciences of the United States of America 108: 16050–5.

Buck BL, Altermann E, Svingerud T and Klaenhammer TR (2005) Functional analysis of putative adhesion factors in Lactobacillus acidophilus NCFM. Applied and Environmental Microbiology 71: 8344–51.

Canani RB, Costanzo MD, Leone L, Bedogni G, Brambilla P, Cianfarani S, Nobili V, Pietrobelli A and Agostoni C (2011) Epigenetic mechanisms elicited by nutrition in early life. Nutrition Research Reviews 24: 198–205.

Cogan TA, Thomas AO, Rees LE, Taylor AH, Jepson MA, Williams PH, Ketley J and Humphrey TJ (2007) Norepinephrine increases the pathogenic potential of Campylobacter jejuni. Gut 56: 1060–5.

Collins SM and Bercik P (2009) The relationship between intestinal microbiota and the central nervous system in normal gastrointestinal function and disease. Gastroenterology 136: 2003–14.

Dantzer R, O'Connor JC, Freund GG, Johnson RW and Kelley KW (2008) From inflammation to sickness and depression: when the immune system subjugates the brain. Nature Reviews Neuroscience 9: 46–56.

Desbonnet L, Garrett L, Clarke G, Bienenstock J and Dinan TG (2008) The probiotic Bifidobacteria infantis: An assessment of potential antidepressant properties in the rat. Journal of Psychiatric Research 43: 164–74.

Diaz Heijtz R, Wang S, Anuar F, Qian Y, Bjorkholm B, Samuelsson A, Hibberd ML, Forssberg H and Pettersson S (2011) Normal gut microbiota modulates brain development and behavior. Proceedings of the National Academy of Sciences of the United States of America 108: 3047–52.

Dinan TG and Cryan JF (2012) Regulation of the stress response by the gut microbiota: implications for psychoneuroendocrinology. Psychoneuroendocrinology 37: 1369–78.

Dotan I and Rachmilewitz D (2005) Probiotics in inflammatory bowel disease: possible mechanisms of action. Current Opinion in Gastroenterology 21: 426–30.

Duncker SC, Wang L, Hols P and Bienenstock J (2008) The D-alanine content of lipoteichoic acid is crucial for Lactobacillus plantarum-mediated protection from visceral pain perception in a rat colorectal distension model. Neurogastroenterology & Motility 20: 843–50.

Forsythe P, Sudo N, Dinan T, Taylor VH and Bienenstock J (2010) Mood and gut feelings. Brain, Behavior, and Immunity 24: 9–16.

Freestone PP, Sandrini S□, Haigh RD and Lyte □ (2008) □icrobial endocrinology: how stress influences susceptibility to infection. Trends in Microbiology 16: 55–64.

Gareau MG, Jury J, MacQueen G, Sherman PM and Perdue MH (2007) Probiotic treatment of rat pups normalises corticosterone release and ameliorates colonic dysfunction induced by maternal separation. Gut 56: 1522–8.

Goehler LE, Gaykema RP, Nguyen KT, Lee JE, Tilders FJ, Maier SF and Watkins LR (1999) Interleukin-1beta in immune cells of the abdominal vagus nerve: a link between the immune and nervous systems? The Journal of Neuroscience 19: 2799–806.

Grenham S, Clarke G, Cryan JF and Dinan TG (2011) Brain–gut-microbe communication in health and disease. Frontiers of Physiology 2: 94.

Guarner F and □alagelada JR (2003) Gut flora in health and disease. Lancet 361: 512–9.

Iyer LM, Aravind L, Coon SL, Klein DC and Koonin EV (2004) Evolution of cell-cell signaling in animals: did late horizontal gene transfer from bacteria have a role? Trends in Genetics 20: 292–9.

Jijon H, Backer J, Diaz H, Yeung H, Thiel D, McKaigney C, De Simone C and Madsen K (2004) DNA from probiotic bacteria modulates murine and human epithelial and immune function. Gastroenterology 126: 1358–73.

Joint FAO/WHO Expert Consultation (2001) Evaluation of Health and Nutritional Properties of Probiotics in Food. ftp://ftp.fao.org/docrep/fao/009/a0512e/a0512e00.pdf Accessed 3 January 2013.

Kankaanpaa PE, Yang B, Kallio HP, Isolauri E and Salminen SJ (2002) Influence of probiotic supplemented infant formula on composition of plasma lipids in atopic infants. Journal of Nutritional Biochemistry 13: 364–369.

Konturek PC, Brzozowski T and Konturek SJ (2011) Stress and the gut: pathophysiology, clinical consequences, diagnostic approach and treatment options. Journal of Physiology and Pharmacology 62: 591–9.

Lan JG, Cruickshank SM, Singh JC, Farrar M, Lodge JP, Felsburg PJ and Carding SR (2005) Different cytokine response of primary colonic epithelial cells to commensal bacteria. World Journal of Gastroenterology 11: 3375–84.

Ley RE, Peterson DA and Gordon JI (2006) Ecological and evolutionary forces shaping microbial diversity in the human intestine. Cell 124: 837–48.

Ma D, Forsythe P and Bienenstock J (2004) Live Lactobacillus rhamnosus [corrected] is essential for the inhibitory effect on tumor necrosis factor alpha-induced interleukin-8 expression. Infection and Immunity 72: 5308–14.

Macpherson AJ and Harris NL (2004) Interactions between commensal intestinal bacteria and the immune system. Nature Reviews Immunology 4: 478–85.

Mai V and Draganov PV (2009) Recent advances and remaining gaps in our knowledge of associations between gut microbiota and human health. World Journal of Gastroenterology 15: 81–5.

Massart R, Mongeau R and Lanfumey L (2012) Beyond the monoaminergic hypothesis: neuroplasticity and epigenetic changes in a transgenic mouse model of depression. Philosophical Transactions of the Royal Society B: Biological Sciences 367: 2485–94.

Metchnikoff E (1907) Lactic acid as inhibiting intestinal putrefaction. pp. 161–183. *In*: E Metchnikoff (ed). The Prolongation of Life: Optimistic studies. W. Heinemann, London.

Montkowski A, Barden N, Wotjak C, Stec I, Ganster J, Meaney M, Engelmann M, Reul JM, Landgraf R and Holsboer F (1995) Long-term antidepressant treatment reduces behavioural deficits in transgenic mice with impaired glucocorticoid receptor function. Journal of Neuroendocrinology 7: 841–5.

Ostman S, Rask C, Wold AE, Hultkrantz S and Telemo E (2006) Impaired regulatory T cell function in germ-free mice. European Journal of Immunology 36: 2336–46.

Rakoff-Nahoum S, Paglino J, Eslami-Varzaneh F, Edberg S and Medzhitov R (2004) Recognition of commensal microflora by toll-like receptors is required for intestinal homeostasis. Cell 118: 229–41.

Rhee SH, Pothoulakis C and Mayer EA (2009) Principles and clinical implications of the brain–gut–enteric microbiota axis. Nature Reviews Gastroenterology & Hepatology 6: 306–14.

Rolls A, Shechter R, London A, Ziv Y, Ronen A, Levy R and Schwartz M (2007) Toll-like receptors modulate adult hippocampal neurogenesis. Nature Cell Biology 9: 1081–8.

Rothenberg ME and Keeffe EB (2005) Antibiotics in the management of hepatic encephalopathy: an evidence-based review. Reviews in Gastroenterological Disorders 3: 26–35.

Rumio C, Besusso D, Arnaboldi F, Palazzo M, Selleri S, Gariboldi S, Akira S, Uematsu S, Bignami P, Ceriani V, Menard S and Balsari A (2006) Activation of smooth muscle and myenteric plexus cells of jejunum via Toll-like receptor 4. Journal of Cellular Physiology 208: 47–54.

Sheil B, McCarthy J, O'Mahony L, Bennett MW, Ryan P, Fitzgibbon JJ, Kiely B, Collins JK, Shanahan F (2004) Is the mucosal route of administration essential for probiotic function? Subcutaneous administration is associated with attenuation of murine colitis and arthritis. Gut 53: 694–700.

Sudo N, Chida Y, Aiba Y, Sonoda J, Oyama N, Yu XN, Kubo C and Koga Y (2004) Postnatal microbial colonization programs the hypothalamic-pituitary-adrenal system for stress response in mice. The Journal of Physiology 558: 263–75.

Sumi Y, □ iyakawa □, Kanzaki □ and Kotake Y (1977) Vitamin B-6 deficiency in germfree rats. Journal of Nutrition 107: 1707–14.

Takeshita Y and Ransohoff R□ (2012) Inflammatory cell trafficking across the blood-brain barrier: chemokine regulation and *in vitro* models. Immunological Reviews 248: 228–39.

Tsankova N, Renthal W, Kumar A and Nestler EJ (2007) Epigenetic regulation in psychiatric disorders. Nature Reviews Neuroscience 8: 355–67.

Turnbaugh PJ, Ley RE, Mahowald MA, Magrini V, Mardis ER and Gordon JI (2006) An obesity-associated gut microbiome with increased capacity for energy harvest. Nature 444: 1027–31.

Ulevitch RJ (1999) Endotoxin opens the Tollgates to innate immunity. Nature Medicine 5: 144–5.

Verdu EF, Bercik P, Verma-Gandhu M, Huang XX, Blennerhassett P, Jackson W, Mao Y, Wang L, Rochat F and Collins S□ (2006) Specific probiotic therapy attenuates antibiotic induced visceral hypersensitivity in mice. Gut 55: 182–90.

Watkins LR and Maier SF (2005) Immune regulation of central nervous system functions: from sickness responses to pathological pain. Journal of Internal Medicine 257: 139–55.

Weaver IC, Cervoni N, Champagne FA, D'Alessio AC, Sharma S, Seckl JR, Dymov S, Szyf M and Meaney MJ (2004) Epigenetic programming by maternal behavior. Nature Neuroscience 7: 847–54.

Wells JM, Rossi O, Meijerink M and van Baarlen P (2011) Epithelial crosstalk at the microbiota-mucosal interface. Proceedings of the National Academy of Sciences of the United States of America 108 Suppl 1: 4607–14.

Woodmansey EJ (2007) Intestinal bacteria and ageing. Journal of Applied Microbiology 102: 1178–86.

CHAPTER 7

Probiotics and Eating Disorders

Ursula Philpot

INTRODUCTION

Eating disorders describe a range of conditions that are defined by abnormal eating habits that involve either inadequate or excessive nutrition to the detriment of an individual's mental and physical health. The most common of these are Binge Eating Disorder, Bulimia Nervosa and Anorexia Nervosa. The aetiology of eating disorders is multifactorial; with psychological, genetic, neurological, and nutritional mechanisms playing a role. The exact biological mechanisms involved in the development or maintenance of these disorders are still poorly understood, but significant alterations in body weight, immunity and gut function are common features across all eating disorders.

The role of probiotics within eating disorders has not been well researched, and their possible mechanisms of influence are not yet well defined. However, the development of emerging theories and a number of significant and interesting smaller studies, make this an exciting new area of study. This chapter focuses on the pathology of body weight, immunity and gut function in eating disorders, exploring the possible role of neuropeptides and discussing the potential role for probiotics in moderating these systems within eating disorders.

Effect of Eating Disorders on Immunity

The wide ranging physical effects of starvation and food restriction are well documented and include: hypothermia, bradycardia, preoccupation with food,

Senior Lecturer, School of Clinical & Applied Sciences, Leeds Beckett University, Leeds, UK.
Email: U.Philpot@leedsbeckett.ac.uk

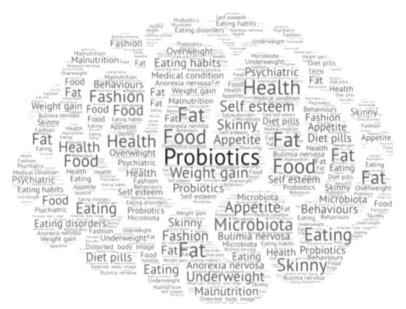

Figure 1

anxiety, poor sleep, gastrointestinal problems and immune system alterations (Kalm and Semba, 2005). Under nutrition due to insufficient macro-nutrients impairs the immune system. Lipids in particular, exert a profound effect in the modulation of the immune system, as the fatty acid composition of lymphocytes and other immune cells is altered according to the fatty acid composition of the diet (Marcos et al., 2003). The most consistent immune abnormalities reported in the literature as a result of under-nutrition are in cell mediated immunity:- specifically phagocytes function (phagocyte cells that protect the body by ingesting harmful foreign particles, bacteria, and dead or dying cells) and cytokines production (cytokine molecules act as hormonal regulators in infection and immune responses). Additionally there are significant alterations to the complement system (molecules found in the blood which are activated in response to infection) and the mucosal secretory antibody response (immunoglobulin's produced in mucosal linings of gastrointestinal tract). The mucosal antibody response has been linked to gut flora and probiotic influence which are discussed later in this chapter.

Hormones have been proposed as key mediators for these abnormalities, with Leptin named as a particularly strong influence. Leptin is a hormone produced by fat cells associated with appetite regulation and energy expenditure and is correlated with BMI in both overweight and underweight individuals. The thymus is a specialized organ of the immune system found in the upper body, which develops immunocompetent T-cells that initiate immune responses following the recognition of pathogens, as well as being self-tolerant (e.g., they are non-reactive to self). The thymus is particularly sensitive to food deprivation and has been designated the "barometer of malnutrition" by Matarase et al., 2000. During starvation, there is a dramatic reduction in Leptin, which appears to link directly to thymus atrophy and in turn immune suppression. Leptin prevents thymic atrophy if administered during starvation in animal models. Further, Leptin replacement during starvation completely protected against starvation induced changes in thymocyte numbers and subpopulation proportions in mice (Matarese et al., 2000). Based on these observations, it has been hypothesized that the decrease in leptin levels that accompanies starvation may contribute to the increased susceptibility to lethal infections that occurs during starvation, particularly the occurrence of asymptomatic or "Silent infections" such as sudden onset pneumonia or Tuberculosis. These are not uncommon in severe and enduring AN, where a reduction in fever response and the signs and symptoms of infection significantly delay diagnosis of such infections and increase the complication rate (Brown et al., 2005).

The direct impact of specific eating disorders on immunity is less well documented. Nonetheless, the research consistently shows significant immune-compromise in anorexia nervosa, in particular leukopenia and lymphocytosis, and delayed hypersensitivity test (Marcos et al., 1993b). In addition, where over exercise is a feature of anorexia nervosa and there is an additional immune system compromise other changes are apparent in the form of altered lymphocyte (white blood cells) counts, delayed hypersensitivity test (DHT) response (an immune function test measuring the presence of activated T cells), and altered cytokine production to stimulus (Nova et al., 2006). It is interesting to note that these finding contrast with reported clinical observations, in which physicians report infrequent episodes of common bacterial and viral infections in patients with Anorexia Nervosa (Marcos, 2000). There may be several explanations for this. Firstly, that in frank starvation there is usually a lack of both macronutrients and micronutrients, whilst in Anorexia Nervosa patients there is a tendency to maintain a high intake of micronutrients via fruit, vegetables and vitamin supplementation, despite inadequate calories. Secondly, mechanism involving modifications in the secretion pattern of pro-inflammatory cytokines could explain some immune function findings in underweight AN patients. Hypothetically, some of the complex interactions occurring between cytokines, the endocrine system and the central nervous system could provide some compensatory mechanisms to adapt to the limited nutrient supply and possibly result in the perceived lack of infection symptoms. A dysregulated cytokine production and the altered acute-phase response to infection, as well as cortisol and leptin, are considered to be potential factors involved in the adaptation processes occurring (Marcos et al., 2003).

Immuno-competency is also strongly influenced by micronutrients. Key nutrients include Vitamin A, Beta-carotene, Vitamin B6 and B12, Vitamin C, Vitamin E, riboflavin, iron, zinc, folic acid, and selenium have all been implicated in altered immune response (Chandra, 2002). For example, antioxidant nutrients play a pivotal role in maintaining the antioxidant/oxidant balance in immune cells and in protecting them from oxidative stress, whilst the addition of the deficient nutrient back to the diet can restore immune function and resistance to infection (Marco et al., 2003). These mechanisms involved are varied and complex.

The effects of Bulimia Nervosa (BN) and Binge eating disorder (BED) on immunity are less well studied. Patients with BN do not become as emaciated as patients with AN, but their weight often fluctuates > 5 kg, due to the alternating binge eating and fasting or purging behaviour. Baseline Leptin level concentration is decreased compared to weight matched controls which may impact on immunity. Significantly leukocyte values have been shown to be lower in BN patients with an illness duration of over 3.5 years, and 40% of the patients have been shown to demonstrate some leukopenia, which in turn is linked to a decrease in most types of white blood cells (Marcos, 1997). In studies of shorter duration (1–1.5 years) no modifications were found in leukocytes, neutrophils, or monocytes, suggesting more severe and enduring patients maybe more immune-compromised (Marcos, 1993a).

Gut Function and Eating Disorders

Functional gastrointestinal disorders (FGID) are common in eating disorder patients, and in the majority of patients these persist even after the recovery from eating disorders, particularly in psychologically distressed patients (Porcelli et al., 1998). Incidence rates are 52% with irritable bowel syndrome (IBS), 51% with functional heartburn (FH), 31% with functional abdominal bloating, at, 24% with functional constipation (FC) and 23% with functional dysphagia. In addition, three or more coexistent FGIDs were found in just over half of all the study population (Boyd, 2005). Psychological variables (somatisation, neuroticism, and anxiety), age and binge eating are significant predictors of FGIDs, but altered eating behaviour is also strongly associated with disturbed gastrointestinal sensitivity and motor physiology. Because FGIDs can persist independently of the outcome of the ED, there has been significant speculation on the mechanisms underlying FGIDs in patients with an ED, and interactions of biological, psychosocial and social factors have all been proposed. Within biological theory, gut microflora have been implicated. Microbiota profiling research demonstrates both quantitative and qualitative changes of mucosal and faecal gut microbiota, particularly where IBS exists as the FGID. The most popular current hypothesis is that abnormal microbiota activate gut mucosal immune responses which increase gut wall permeability, activate nerve cell sensory pathways, and deregulate the guts nervous system (Simrén et al., 2012).

Neuropeptide Role in Development and Maintenance of Eating Disorders

Neuropeptides are small protein-like molecules (peptides) used by neurons to communicate with each other. These neuronal signalling molecules influence the activity of the brain in specific ways, and are involved in a wide range of brain functions including reward system activation, food intake, metabolism, reproduction, social behaviours, learning and memory.

Neuropeptides may well have a significant part to play in the pathogenesis of eating disorders. A small, but noteworthy body of research indicates that alterations of central and/or peripheral neuropeptidergic signalling are accompanied by disturbed regulation of body weight, appetite, or emotion (Benoit et al., 2008; Hofbauer et al., 2008; Fetissov et al., 2008).

Substances called autoantibodies may also play a significant role here. An autoantibody is an antibody that reacts against normal substances present in the organism, and is commonly found in autoimmune diseases. AutoAbs directed against stress related hormones: alpha-melanocyte-stimulating hormone (α-MSH—a neuropeptide that helps to regulate appetite and emotion) and adrenocorticotrophic hormone (ACTH) are higher in patients with eating disorders compared with controls. Fetissov and colleagues (2008) found that the level of one of these autoantibodies (AutoAbs α-MSH) was directly correlated with higher scores of restrictive eating behaviour as measured by the Eating Disorders Inventory-2 (Garner, 1991). They also found significant linear (positive and negative) correlations between autoAbs directed against four other key neuropeptides (ACTH, α-MSH, Oxytocin, Vasopressin) in patients with AN and BN. Data from other studies supports the finding that levels of AutoAbs are altered in different ways in AN compared to obesity (Kalra, 2008). There is also growing support for this theory from animal models, for example intracerebral injection of α-MSH IgA autoABs in rat models produces acute bulimic and anxious responses (Lee et al., 2008; Fetissov et al., 2008).

Although the mechanisms underlying the alterations in α-MSH autoAB production in the development of eating disorders has not been identified, gut microflora appears as a likely target, both for autoAb production, and their modulation. Theory by Fetissov and Dechelotte (2011) suggest that a process of "molecular mimicry" takes places between microbial and self-proteins, e.g., the same sequence for 5 or more amino acids appearing in appetite regulating proteins, also appear in microbes commonly found in the body, e.g., Candia albicans and Helicobacter pylori. The microbial proteins present these mimicked amino acid sequences to Peyers patches (aggregations of lymphoid tissue that are usually found in the lowest portion of the small intestine) or other lymphoid organs. This stimulates the production of immunoglobulins that bind to the identical region in the endogenous regulatory peptides, and so modulate hormone signalling pathways.

Whilst gut microflora is not compulsory for the presence of neuropeptide autoABs, it appears it can modulate levels of some of the autoABs. For example, production of IgA is an important adaptation to the presence of beneficial intestinal bacteria. The presence of IgA class of neuropeptides autoAbs suggests that at least some of these autoAbs can be stimulated by luminal antigens including microbial proteins of the gut microflora (Macpherson, 2007). Induction of the response is localised within the intestinal mucosal immune system. This compartmentalization allows a vigorous mucosal immune response without needing the systemic immune system to be tolerant of these organisms.

To conclude: In normal circumstances, helpful (commensual) gut microflora participate in the production of AutoAbs cross-reacting with regulatory peptides by the presentation of proteins of a similar structure. It is proposed that these autoABs maintain a balance between the biological effects exerted by a corresponding peptide on its specific receptors, and clearance of peptides by degradation, resulting in maintenance of energy and emotional homeostasis. In contrast, pathogenic gut microflora may stimulate production of pathogenic peptide-reactive autoABs that will alter the normal balance between biological activity and the clearance of regulatory peptides, possibly resulting in eating disorders and other neurological disorders (Fetissov et al., 2008).

The Role of Gut Microflora in Body Weight Regulation

The gut microflora is now a fairly well established environmental regulator of fat storage and adiposity, with short chain fatty acid production and low grade inflammation suggested as underlying mechanisms of action (Musso et al., 2010; Armougom et al., 2009). Experimental data in animals, and observational studies in obese patients, suggest that the composition of the gut microbiota differs in obese and lean individuals, and in patients presenting with other diseases associated with obesity or nutritional dysfunction, such as non-alcoholic steatohepatitis. Armougom and colleagues (2009) monitored gut bacteria in patients of a range of weights, and found that there were significant differences between lean, obese and anorexic patients. Patients with Anorexia Nervosa had much higher levels of Methangens, specifically M. smithii. These are involved in the removal of hydrogen excess from the human gut, reducing it to methane and allowing for an increase in the transformation of nutrients into calories (Ley et al., 2006). This increase in Methangens may be explained as a possible adaptive response to chronic low calorie diet in AN where M. smithii recycles hydrogen in methane, allowing for an increase in the transformation of nutrients into calories, or as a response to constipation found in AN, where an increase in methane producing-bacteria has been demonstrated (Armougom et al., 2009).

Recent studies have looked at the effects of modulating gut microflora to modify weight gain (Mekkes et al., 2013). Lactobacillus, the most dominant microflora found in obese subjects, has been proposed as a possible aid to weight gain. This theory has some support from animal studies (Khan et al., 2007), and appears to be an interesting area of future development within eating disorders. Conversely, in animal studies, the ingestion of dietary fibres with prebiotic properties, and treatment with antibiotics results in an improvement in the metabolic abnormalities associated with obesity. This suggests that these microbial strains can be applied in the treatment of obesity; thereby establishing gut microbiota as a realistic therapeutic target in the future for conditions which involve weight management (Mekkes et al., 2013). Further research should be directed to the most effective combination and dosage rate of probiotic microorganisms.

Role of Probiotics in Managing FGID's

The etiology of irritable bowel syndrome (IBS) is thought to be multifactorial, with several factors including alterations in gut motility, bacterial overgrowth, microscopic inflammation, and visceral hypersensitivity potentially playing a role. The balance of normal gut microflora is significant. For example, bacterial or viral gastroenteritis can sometimes lead to chronic IBS symptoms that may continue long after recovery from the initial sickness, known as post-infectious IBS, which is associated with symptoms of abdominal pain/discomfort, diarrhoea and abdominal bloating, gas, and distension. Small-intestinal bacterial overgrowth, where the increase in bacteria in the small intestines can lead to increased fermentation of undigested sugars, resulting in excessive gas production and changes in the motility of the GI tract, responds well to antibiotic treatment decreasing the amount of bacteria in the small intestines.

Data on the effects of probiotics in functional GI disorders is still limited. Early studies in functional bowel disorders were small and had methodological limitations, leading to inconsistent results; in the last few years researchers have begun to accumulate more significant data on the use of probiotic in patients with these disorders. The results of these studies have shown that daily supplementation of diet with certain probiotics can improve intestinal physiology, such as increase intestinal transit time and improve symptoms such as bloating, gas, and discomfort. Probiotic treatments are therefore recommended as adjunctive treatment modalities for IBS in mainstream guidance (McKenzie et al., 2012).

It is proposed that probiotics may also modulate hormone signalling in the gut. There is some limited support for this theory from animal models. Gut microflora influence the release of peptides and play a role in regulating gastrointestinal endocrine cells (Forsythe et al., 2012). Little is known about the effect of probiotics on the expression and release of hormonal components of gut/brain communication. However, gut microbiota can alter nutrient availability, and there is a close relationship between nutrient sensing and peptide secretion by gastric cells. Most research studies examining the role of probiotics in IBS are small in size and of short duration. Larger, well-controlled studies are needed to help establish the most effective probiotic dose and duration of therapy; whether there is a role for maintenance of IBS therapy or only IBS therapy on an as-needed basis. In addition, cost-effectiveness analysis and safety profiles still need to be addressed in large, well-designed trials.

Probiotics to Support Immunity in Eating Disorders

The numbers of studies that have looked at the role of probiotics in eating disorders are small. Studies have mainly been undertaken in adolescent populations, have been of short duration, and contained design flaws. However, they do provide interesting insight into potential role for probiotics in supporting immune function in this patient population.

In their 2006 paper, the effects of nutritional intervention with yogurt on lymphocyte subsets and cytokine production capacity in Anorexia Nervosa, Nova et al., 2006 proposed that the addition of natural yogurt to the diets of adolescent patients with AN who were undergoing a process of refeeding, would enhance immune function. A small group of 16 patients with AN and 16 healthy controls consumed yogurt containing 10^7–10^8 cfu per ml of Lactobacillus delbrueckii and Streptococcus thermophulis (375 grams per day) for 10 weeks. As a control, 14 patients with AN and 19 healthy adolescents consumed milk (400 ml per day) for the same time-period. Because both increased nutrition, and weight gain would positively impact on immune function, the researchers were looking for a significant difference in specific white blood cells between the AN group taking milk, compared to the AN group taking yogurt. Dairy consumption in all groups was well controlled. This study looked at the ratio of two types of white blood cells—CD4+ and CD8+. The studies demonstrated significant differences in CD4+/CD8+ ratio and in IFN-Y production between the milk and yogurt group. These results support the inclusion of Yogurt in refeeding of anorexia nervosa patients highlighting a potential positive effect on immunological markers of immunity, specifically CD4+/CD8+ ratio, and IFN-Y production by lymphocytes.

In a similar study looking at the effect of fermented milk on interferon production in Anorexia Nervosa patients, Solis and colleagues (2002) also looked to support the theory that adding yogurt to the refeeding regimen of patients with anorexia nervosa could lead to enhanced INF-Y production. A randomised cross over design was used with 27 patients randomly assigned to two groups. One group consumed 375 g Yogurt daily, and the other 450 g milk daily, after a 10-week period the groups crossed and consumed the alternate product. The results showed a significant positive association with increased IFN-Y production in association with yogurt consumption in both groups. Interestingly the stimulatory effect on IFN-Y production occurred only after 10 weeks, and not at the start of consumption, suggesting the need for continuous treatment.

Haruta et al. (2012) present an interesting case report of an acutely ill patient with Anorexia Nervosa, who among other problems developed a severe bacterial infection on refeeding. The case discusses the atrophy of the intestinal mucosa and consequent bacterial translocation as a cause of the infection, and the treatment with both antibiotics and lactic acid bacterial probiotics, and glutamine alongside prebiotics of oligosaccharides and fibre. This again lends support to the role of probiotics in maintaining gut integrity, and function in eating disorders.

To summarise. There is very limited research in the area of probiotics and eating disorders, although strong theoretical models exist based on animal and human studies. Theory suggests a possible role for probiotics in both the development and recovery from eating disorders, specifically through neuropeptide modulation, and the action of probiotics on immunity, gut function and body weight.

Future research opportunities should focus on increasing our understanding of the complex interplay play between the gut, the immune system, the endocrine system and the nutritional system that contribute to the development and maintenance of eating disorders. This will support the identification of potential new Probiotics treatments and help to develop more robust data around the type, dose and optimal treatments approaches for sufferers of eating disorders.

References

Armougom F, Henry M, Vialettes B, Raccah D and Raoult D (2009) Monitoring bacterial community of human gut microbiota reveals an increase in Lactobacillus in obese patients and Methanogens in Anorexic Patients 4.

Benoit S, Tracy A, Davis J and Choi D (2008) Novel functions of orexigenic hypothalamic peptides: From genes to behaviour. Nutrition 24: 843–7.

Boyd C, Abraham S and Kellow J (2005) Psychological features are important predictors of functional gastrointestinal disorders in patients with eating disorders. Scandinavian Journal of Gastroenterology 40: 929–935.

Brown RF, Bartrop R, Beumont P and Birmingham CL (2005) Bacterial infections in anorexia nervosa: delayed recognition increases complications. International Journal of Eating Disorders 37: 261–5.

Chandra RK (2002) Nutrition and the immune system from birth to old age. European Journal Clinical Nutrition 56: 73–76.

Fetissov S, Hamze Sinno M, Coquerel Q, Do Rego J, Coëffier M, Gilbert t, Hökfelt T and Déchelotte P (2008) Emerging role of autoantibodies against appetite-regulating neuropeptides in eating disorders. Nutrition 24: 854–859.

Fetissov S and Dechelotte P (2011) The link between gut–brain axis and neuropsychiatric disorders. Current Opinion in Clinical Nutrition and Metabolic Care 14: 477–482.

Forsythe P, Kunze WA and Bienenstock J (2012) On communication between gut microbes and the brain. Curr. Opin. Gastroenterol. 28: 557–562. 10.1097/MOG.0b013e3283572ff.

Garner DM (1991) Eating Disorder Inventory-2 professional manual. Odessa, FL: Psychological Assessment Resources.

Haruta I, Asakawa A, Ogiso K, Amitani H, Amitani M, Tsai M, Hamada S and Inui A (2012) A case of anorexia nervosa with disseminated intravascular coagulation Syndrome. International Journal of Eating Disorders 45:3 453–455.

Hofbauer K, Lecourt A and Peter J (2008) Antibodies as pharmacological tools for studies on the regulation of energy balance. Nutrition 24: 791–7.

Kalm L and Semba R (2005) They starved so that others be better fed: remembering ancel keys and the minnesota experiment. Journal Nutrition 135: 1347–1352.

Kalra SP (2008) Disruptions in the leptin-NPY link underlies the pandemic of diabetes and metabolic syndrome: new therapeutic approaches. Nutrition 24: 820–6.

Lee N, Enriquez R, Boey D, Lin, Slack K, Baldock P, Herzog H and Sainsbury A (2008) Synergistic attenuation of obesity by Y2- and Y4-receptor double knockout in ob/ob mice. Nutrition 24: 892–9.

Ley RE, Turnbaugh P, Klein S and Gordon J (2006) Human gut microbes associated with obesity. Nature 444: 1022–1023 (21 December 2006).

Macpherson AJ and Slack E (2007) The functional interactions of commensal bacteria with intestinal secretory IgA. Current Opinion Gastroenterology 23: 673–8.

Marcos A, Varela P, Santacruz I and Muhoz-Velez A (1993a) Evaluation of immunocompetence and nutritional status in patients with Bulimia Nervosa. American Journal Clinical Nutrition 57: 65.

Marcos A, Varela P, Santacruz I, Munoz-Vela A and Morande G (1993b) Nutritional status and immune-competence in eating disorders. A comparative study. European Journal Clinical Nutrition 47: 787–793.

Marcos A (1997) The immune system in eating disorders: an overview. Current Concepts in Nutrition. Nutrition, Immunology, Neuroscience, and Behaviour: Part VII Number 10.

Marcos A (2000) Eating disorders: a situation of malnutrition and peculiar changes in the immune system. European Journal of Clinical Nutrition 54: S61–64.

Marcos A, Nova E and Montero A (2003) Changes in the immune system are conditioned by nutrition. European Journal of Clinical Nutrition 57, Suppl 1: S66–S69.

Matarase G (2000) Leptin and the immune system; how nutritional status influences the immune response. European Cytokine Network 11: 7–13.

McKenzie Y, Alder A, Anderson A, Willis A, Goddard L, Gulia P, Jankovich E, Mutch P, Reeves L, Singer A and Lomer M (2012) British dietetic association evidence-based guidelines for the dietary management of irritable bowel syndrome in adults. Journal of Human Nutrition and Dietetics 260–274.

Mekkes M, Weenen T, Brummer R and Claassen E (2013) The development of probiotic treatment in obesity: a review. Journal of Beneficial Microbes 1–10.

Musso G, Gambino R and Cassader M (2010) The hygiene hypothesis expanded? Obesity, diabetes, and gut microbiota. Diabetes Care 33(10): 2277–2284.

Nova E et al. (2006) Effects of a nutritional intervention with yogurt on lymphocyte subsets and cytokine production capacity in anorexia nervosa patients. European Journal of Nutrition 45(4): 225–233.

Porcelli P, Leandro G and De Carne M (1998) Functional gastrointestinal disorders and eating disorders: relevance of the association in clinical management. Scandinavian Journal of Gastroenterology 33(6): 577–582 (doi:10.1080/00365529850171819).

Simrén M, Barbara G, Flint H, Spiegel B, Spiller R, Vanner S, Verdu E, Whorwell P and Zoetendal E (2012) Intestinal microbiota in functional bowel disorders: a Rome foundation report. Gut Gut published online June 22 2012.

Solis B, Nova E, Gomez S, Samartı´ S, Mouane N, Lemtouni A, Belaoui H and Marcos A (2002) The effect of fermented milk on interferon production in malnourished children and in anorexia nervosa patients undergoing nutritional care. European Journal of Clinical Nutrition 56, Suppl 4: S27–S33.

CHAPTER 8

Probiotics and Obsessive-Compulsive Disorder

Derek Larkin[1,]* and *Colin R Martin*[2]

INTRODUCTION

Obsessive-compulsive disorder (OCD) is a debilitating chronic condition characterized by intrusive, ego dystonic ideas or impulses that often accompany ritualistic and time-consuming compulsions (Rees, 2014). The obsessions and compulsions can be extremely diverse, and the assessment and rating of the OCD symptoms to establish severity of the disorder are complex due to the nature of the disorder itself (Zohar, 2012).

OCD first came to light in the 17th century, a time in which obsessions were considered to exist purely within a religious framework, therefore individuals with obsessions were thought to be possessed by outside forces, such as the devil. Individuals, with compulsive behaviours were quite often treated with the method of exorcism (Menzies and De Silva, 2003). One of the first fictional portrayals of OCD is in Shakespeare's illustration of Lady Macbeth in which she attempts to rid herself of guilt by repeatedly engaging in hand washing (Menzies and De Silva, 2003).

The estimated lifetime prevalence of OCD is 1.2 to 1.8%, and is generally thought to have significant impairments to quality-of-life in both the patient and the immediate family (Kugler et al., 2013; Eisen et al., 2006; APA, 2013). There are often very limited treatment regimens offered to OCD patients, which mainly consist of pharmacotherapy, and generally various forms of cognitive behavioural intervention (Abudy et al., 2011). The first line of the intervention generally involves

[1] Edge Hill University, St Helens Road, Ormsirk, Lancashire, L39 4QP.
[2] Faculty of Society and Health, Buckinghamshire New University, Uxbridge Campus, 106 Oxford Road, Uxbridge, Middlesex, UB8 1NA, UK.
* Corresponding author

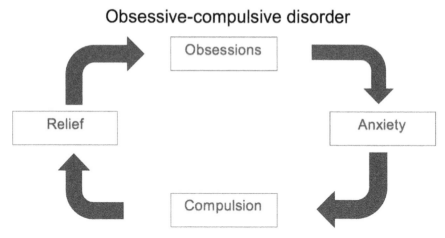

Figure 1 OCD response mechanism.

the administration of selective serotonin reuptake inhibitors (SSRI) but the evidence seems to suggest that patients with OCD do not generally respond well to this line of treatment, and there is an argument that the use of SSRI's in OCD is palliative at best (Rees, 2014).

In recent years there has been major interest in exploring the links between the health of the gut and mental health (Schmidt, 2015). Three pathways have been identified that describe how gut microbiota may influence mental health, through inflammation, the hypothalamic-pituitary-adrenal axis (HPA), or interference with neurotransmitter signalling (Uher and McGuffin, 2010). Increased activity in the HPA axis has been reported in OCD. In general terms the HPA axis and the sympathetic nervous system mediate concentrations of the stress hormones adrenaline, noradrenaline and cortisol (de Kloet et al., 2005). Increased activity in the HPA axis has been noted in OCD patients were increased levels of corticotrophin releasing hormone, adrenocorticotrophic hormone has been detected in OCD patient's relative to normal controls (Altemus et al., 1992; Catapano et al., 1992). Evidence is starting to show that the HPA axis is sensitive to gut microbiota, and that the manipulation of gut microbiota can in turn alter HPA responses (Zimomra et al., 2011). A handful of studies have starting to emerge indicating that probiotics can mediate some of the symptoms of OCD.

Obsessive-Compulsive Disorder

According to the Diagnostic and Statistical Manual of Mental Disorders (DSM-5, APA, 2013) obsessive-compulsive and related disorders include obsessive-compulsive disorder, body dysmorphic disorder, hoarding disorder, trichotillomania (hair pulling disorder), excoriation (skin-picking) disorder, substance/medication induced obsessive-compulsive and related disorder, obsessive compulsive and related disorder due to other medical conditions and other specified excessive compulsive and related disorders and unspecified obsessive-compulsive and related disorders (e.g., body focused repetitive behaviour disorder, obsessional jealousy) are categorized under the general heading of obsessive-compulsive and related disorders. The DSM-5 characterizes OCD as the presence of obsessions and/or compulsions. Obsessions can be current and persistent thoughts, urges, or images that are experienced as intrusive and unwanted. Whereas compulsions are repetitive behaviours or mental acts that an individual feel's driven to perform in response to an obsession according to rules that must be applied rigidly. The DSM goes on to describe how some obsessive-compulsive and related disorders are characterized by preoccupations by repetitive behaviours or mental acts in response to preoccupations. The obsessions and compulsions vary enormously between individuals; however certain commonalities exist including those of cleaning (contamination obsession and cleaning compulsions); symmetry (symmetry obsessions and repeating, ordering and counting compulsion) forbidden or taboos thoughts (for example aggressive sexual and religious obsessions and related compulsions) and harm (e.g., fear of harm to oneself or others and related checking compulsions) (APA, 2013). Obsessions are often time-consuming and can cause clinically significant distress or impairment in social, occupational, or other important areas of life. OCD is often an indicator of other conditions such as body dysmorphic disorder or general anxiety disorder (APA, 2013). The prevalence of OCD is thought to be around 1.1 to 1.8% and does not differ fundamentally internationally. Suicidal thoughts occur in as many as 50% of individuals with OCD (APA, 2013). OCD is associated with reduced quality-of-life as well as a reduced level of social and occupational attainment. Many individuals with OCD will have impairments because of the time spent obsessing and carrying out compulsions and avoiding situations that can trigger obsessive compulsion that can also severely restrict functioning (APA, 2013).

There are only two treatment modalities that have been shown to be effective in treating OCD symptomatology: (1) cognitive behavioural therapy (CBT) primarily used as a behavioural prevention intervention and (2) pharmacological treatment with selective serotonin reuptake inhibitors (SSRIs). In most cases there is a combination of both interventions (Coyne et al., 2007). Cognitive behavioural treatment has the advantages of apparent durability of treatment effects and the avoidance of potential side effects of medication. CBT can be extremely effective however, if a fast response is needed. Medication may be the initial treatment method if there are concerns with urgency, expense and anxiety associated with behavioural treatment. Over the past few decades' studies have reported that SSRIs can be extremely effective in treating OCD symptoms in young children and adolescents. There are a number of pharmacological interventions that are somewhat routinely prescribed; clomipramine in young children, fluoxetine in children aged eight years and older, sertraline in children six years and older, paroxetine in adults and fluvoxamine in children aged eight years and older (Coyne et al., 2007).

Gut Brain Axis

The link between the brain and gut has recently gained much attention. This complex interplay between the brain and the gut, integrates neural, hormonal and immunological signalling, involving the central nervous system (CNS) and the enteric nervous system (ENS) (Collins et al., 2012). Turna et al. (2015) has stated that there appears to be top-down modulation of gastrointestinal function by stress and emotion as well as a bottom up signalling from visceral afferents to the brain in abdominal pain symptoms and emotional regulation. Published research tends to show that emotional factors such as stress and depression can influence chronic conditions of gastrointestinal illnesses by the brain gut axis (Cryan and Dinan, 2012).

The microbiota has been strongly implicated in the onset and progression of a number of conditions such as inflammatory bowel disease (ulcerative colitis and Crohn's disease), and irritable bowel syndrome (Morgan et al., 2012), autism (Parracho et al., 2005) coeliac disease (Nadal et al., 2007), diabetes (Brown et al., 2011) and obesity (Turnbaugh et al., 2006). Crucially many of these conditions have also been associated with psychiatric comorbidities such as anxiety and depression (Collins et al., 2012; Turna et al., 2015). Over the past few decades there has been major interest in exploring the link between the health of the gut and mental health (Schmidt, 2015). A number of routes have been identified that describe how gut microbiota may influence depression, and related conditions; through inflammation, the hypothalamic-pituitary-adrenal axis (HPA), or interference with neurotransmitter signalling (Uher and McGuffin, 2010). Gut bacteria maybe a pathway that could be exploited to develop novel interventions, to help mitigate some of the major symptoms of inflammatory bowel conditions and targeted psychiatric comorbidities.

Numerous bacteria live in the human gut, generally referred to as gut microbiome, in which they facilitate nutrient absorption by metabolizing indigestible dietary compounds such as gut-associated lymphoid tissue, and by producing vitamins and preventing colonization of pathogens (Rees, 2014). Under normal circumstances the gut microbiome is relatively stable (Faith et al., 2013) but this delicate balance can be compromised by infection, antibiotics and probiotics (Turna et al., 2015). Research has shown that dysfunction of gut microbiome can have an impact on chronic and acute diseases (Turna et al., 2015).

In recent years' interest, has started to grow which has begun to explore the relationship between gut microbiome and the onset and progression of several psychiatric disorders (Naseribafrouei et al., 2014; Jiang et al., 2015). These two studies explored possible differences between the gut microbiome by evaluating differences in terms of species diversity and abundance of operational taxonomic units between depressed in healthy individuals (Turna et al., 2015). Naseribafrouei et al. (2014) found no relationship in terms of species abundance or species diversity, but they did find a difference at the domain level in which *Bacteroides* were underrepresented in the gut microbiota of depressed individuals. This finding is rather confusing as *Bacteroides* species are significant clinical pathogens and are found in most anaerobic infections (Wexler, 2007) therefore an increase in *Bacteroides* would have been expected. Other studies (Jiang et al., 2015) found that individuals with major depressive disorder showed increased faecal microbial diversity, presented with increased levels of *Bacteroides* and *Proteobacteria* while the *Firmicutes* population was significantly decreased. The differences in the findings may have been a product of different methodologies and sample groups. However, there is an increasing pool of evidence which tends to recognise the influential connection between the psychiatric disorders and gut microbiome. There is thought to be a bi-direction and indirect pathway between the brain and the gut. Four candidates have been identified; production of neurotransmitters (Turna et al., 2015), activating gut hormones release from enteroendocrine cells (Collins et al., 2012; Cryan and Dinan, 2012), activation of the enteric nervous system and signalling of the brain via ascending neural pathways (Crumeyrolle-Arias et al., 2014; Turna et al., 2015). And lastly immune activation via cytokines release through mucosal immune cells (Collins et al., 2012; Cryan and Dinan, 2012).

There are several gut bacteria known to release neurotransmitter implicated in psychiatric disorders *Candida*, *Streptococcus*, *Escherichia*, and *Enterococcus* are known to release serotonin, *Bacillus*, and *Serratia* are known to produce Dopamine, *Lactobacillus, Bifidobacterium* are known to produce γ-aminobutyric acid (GABA), *Escherichia*, *Bacillus*, and *Saccharomyces* produces norepinephrine, and *Lactobacillus* produces acetylcholine. It is thought that the produced neurotransmitter in the gut may induce epithelial cells to release molecules that modulate neural signalling within the enteric nervous system, or they may act within a direct pathway on afferent axons (Turna et al., 2015).

Stress has gained the greatest level of attention in relation to microbiota and central nervous system functioning. Hypothalamic-pituitary-adrenal (HPA), axis and its relationship within the stress response, and the effect on microbiota has long been established (Lyte, 2011). A number of rodent studies have established that maternal separation, crowding, heat and acoustic stress have all been found to have a negative impact on microbiota composition (Turna et al., 2015). The HPA axis is a neuro-endocrine response to stress, but also to mood disorders and functional disease (Naseribafrouei et al., 2014). Adjustments to the HPA axis have been observed in individuals with various mental health conditions, including post-traumatic stress disorder, schizophrenia, social anxiety and depression (Naseribafrouei et al., 2014). Research using rodents has found that probiotics are able to interfere with the HPA axis response to acute physiological stress and according to Naseribafrouei et al. (2014) this would indicate a mechanistic connection linking the gut microbiota, HPA and stress. Evidence is mounting, at least in the animal model, that shows an enhanced HPA axis response in germ free (GF) mice to psychological stressors, which provides the idea that gut microbiome has a role in programming the stress response (Sudo et al., 2004; Turna et al., 2015). The way in which these mechanisms work, for the stress-induced activation of the immune system and the HPA axis, has been described as a 'leaky gut' (increased bacterial translocation) (Maes et al., 2012; Maes et al., 2013). It is argued that there is an increased translocation of gut bacteria due to a compromised gut barrier. The gut is thought to have become compromised as a result of either stress or microbiota dysbiosis, in which translocated metabolites directly interact with immune cells (Turna et al., 2015). It has been proposed that intestinal permeability results in increase circulation of bacterial derived lipopolysaccharide that trigger immunological and inflammatory response characterize by increased systemic levels of pro-inflammatory cytokines (Qin et al., 2007; Turna et al., 2015). Maes et al. (2012); Maes et al. (2013) observed the translocation of gut bacteria in patients with depression, Severance et al. (2013) reported a similar finding in a schizophrenic population. The leaky aspects of the gut can be modulated by the administration of probiotics (Ait-Belgnaoui et al., 2012; Savignac et al., 2014).

Obsessive-Compulsive Disorder and Probiotics

There is a distinct lack of research concerning obsessive compulsive disorder (OCD) and the use of probiotics. One of the few studies was conducted by Kantak et al. (2014). Kantak et al. (2014) used *Lactobacillus rhamnosus GG* in mice, to induce OCD type behaviours, the mice were administered RU24960, which is a 5HT (serotonin)$_{1A/1B}$ receptor agonist. RU24960 and similar compounds have been reported to induce anxiogenic responses in rats and mice (Griebel, 1995; Pellow et al., 1987). It has also been reported that 5HT$_{1B}$ receptor agonists also aggravate OCD symptoms in humans (Shanahan et al., 2011). Kantak et al. (2014) pre-treated mice with either a probiotic or a neutral substance for 2–54 weeks, after which OCD like behaviours were induced by the administration of RU24960, they report that marble burying and locomotor behaviour was significantly attenuated in mice treated with the probiotic compared to control mice. In a subsequent study a third group of mice were introduced, and were pre-treated for 4 weeks with fluoxetine, first line treatment for OCD. Kantak et al. (2014) report that both groups pre-treated with fluoxetine and probiotic showed significant reduction in OCD like behaviours. Messaoudi et al. (2011a) demonstrated that in the general population *Lactobacillus helveticus* R0052 and *Bifidobacterium logum* R0175 taken in combination for just 30 days decreases global scores on the hospital anxiety and depression scale (HADs) and the global severity index of the Hopkins symptoms checklist (HSCL-90). This finding was mainly as a result of decreases in the subscales related to somatization, depression and anger hostility domains. In a follow-up analysis Messaoudi et al. (2011b) found that the administration of *Lactobacillus helveticus* and *Bifidobacterium logum* also appears to reduce obsessive-compulsive scores on the Hopkins symptom checklist. Drawing a general conclusion from the evidence so far, it would seem reasonable to suggest that deregulation of the micro-bacteria in the gut may be involved in OCD. Although this observation is only speculative, hypothetically OCD can be explained by communication between the microbiome, inflammation response, and the HPA axis (Turna et al., 2015).

An increasing number of studies appear to show that inflammation processes due to an acute or chronic infection or post-infectious immune response may be involved in the pathogenesis of obsessive-compulsive disorder.

Around 15 years ago the first cases of paediatric autoimmune neuropsychiatric disorder associated with streptococcal infection (PANDAS) were described. Since this time research has been divided between studies that successfully demonstrate an etiologic relationship between streptococcal infections, and childhood-onset obsessive-compulsive disorder, and studies which have not found an association (Swedo et al., 2015). PANDAS is characterized by acute exacerbation of OCD like symptom, which may also include motor/phonic tics following a prodromal group Aβ-haemolytic streptococcal infection (Turna et al., 2015). Even though there is still controversy in relation to the aetiology of PANDAS there appears to be a clinical overlap between PANDAS and OCD type symptoms and pure OCD, which appear to suggest a common aetiological mechanism (Swedo, 2010). However other studies have found different aetiologies and associated OCD with infections such as Borna virus disease (Dietrich et al., 2005). Borna disease virus is a unique virus with a non-segmented, single-stranded RNA-genome of negative polarity and causes behavioural disturbances in animals (Hornig et al., 2001). The process by which Borna disease virus impacts on behavioural and neurophysiological disturbances in OCD is however unknown. Toxoplasma encephalitis is a common presentation of Toxoplasma gondii infection of the central nervous system. The most commonly affected central nervous region in Toxoplasma gondii is the cerebral hemisphere, followed by the basal ganglia, cerebellum and brainstem. The basal ganglia have been implicated in the development of OCD. Miman et al. (2010) found the presence of increased levels of IgC antibodies to Toxoplasma gondii in OCD patients when compared to levels in healthy controls. They conclude that there appears to be causal relationship between chronic toxoplasmosis and the aetiology of OCD. It would seem from the evidence presented that there could be a connection between the immune system and development of OCD.

Conclusion

There are very few treatment methods for OCD, and those that are used are less than ideal because of the potential side-effects, this is complicated by the unclear pathophysiology and aetiology of OCD. There is however an increasing evidence base which suggests that the gut microbiome and gut brain interaction may play an important role in the development and progression of psychiatric disorders. Many studies appear to show a clear link between potential alterations of this axis or changes made to this axis that influence behaviour, this is particularly well-defined in relation to mood and anxiety disorders. Potential treatment modalities that affect gut microbiome, and the gut brain interaction may be more effective means of treatment than many psychiatric illnesses which may include OCD. Research into exploring potential treatment modalities is in its infancy, consequently there is a need for further studies. Current research mainly based on animal models although supplemented with some human data appears to suggest the administration of specific strains of probiotics may moderate OCD type behaviours. There could be an argument which suggests that the first line of OCD treatments may include selective serotonin reuptake inhibitors supplemented with cognitive behavioural therapy, and the administration of gut flora therapy. Turna et al. (2015) also suggest that if a disruption in microbiome can be established in OCD, then this leaves the door open for treatments such as antibiotics, probiotics and faecal biotherapy. This clearly needs further investigation but could serve as a catalyst for a new direction of OCD research leading to potential treatments.

References

Abudy A, Juven-Wetzler A and Zohar J (2011) Pharmacological management of treatment-resistant obsessive-compulsive disorder. CNS Drugs 25: 585–596.

Ait-Belgnaoui A, Durand H, Cartier C, Chaumaz G, Eutamene H, Ferrier L, Houdeau E, Fioramonti J, Bueno L and Theodorou V (2012) Prevention of gut leakiness by a probiotic treatment leads to attenuated HPA response to an acute psychological stress in rats. Psychoneuroendocrinology 37: 1885–1895.

Altemus M, Pigott T, Kalogeras KT, Demitraack M, Dubbert B, Murphy DL and Gold PW (1992) Abnormalities in the regulation of vasopressin and corticotropin releasing factor secretion in obsessive-compulsive disorder. Archives of General Psychiatry 49: 9–20.

APA (2013) Diagnostic and Statistical Manual of Mental Disorders 5th Edition, Washington, DC: American Psychiatric Association.

Brown CT, Davis-Richardson AG, Giongo A, Gano KA, Crabb DB, Mukherjee N, Casella G, Drew JC, Ilonen J, Knip M, Hyoty H, Veijola R, Simell T, Simell O, Neu J, Wasserfall CH, Schatz D, Atkinson MA and Triplett EW (2011) Gut microbiome metagenomics analysis suggests a functional model for the development of autoimmunity for type 1 diabetes. PloS One 6: e25792.

Catapano F, Monteleone P, Fuschino A, Maj M and Kemali D (1992) Melatonin and cortisol secretion in patients with primary obsessive-compulsive disorder. Psychiatry Research 44: 217–225.

Collins SM, Surette M and Bercik P (2012) The interplay between the intestinal microbiota and the brain. Nature Reviews Microbiology 10: 735–742.

Coyne L, Freeman J and Garcia A (2007) Obsessive-compulsive disorder in children. *In*: Gabbard GO (Ed.). Gabbard's Treatments of Psychiatric Disorders. Washington DC: American Psychiatric Publishing. Inc.

Crumeyrolle-Arias M, Jaglin M, Bruneau A, Vancassel S, Cardona A, Dauge V, Naudon L and Rabot S (2014) Absence of the gut microbiota enhances anxiety-like behavior and neuroendocrine response to acute stress in rats. Psychoneuroendocrinology 42: 207–217.

Cryan JF and Dinan TG (2012) Mind-altering microorganisms: the impact of the gut microbiota on brain and behaviour. Nature Reviews Neuroscience 13: 701–712.

de Kloet ER, Joels M and Holsboer F (2005) Stress and the brain: from adaptation to disease. Nature Reviews: Neuroscience 6: 463–475.

Dietrich D, Zhang Y, Bode L, Munte TF, Hauser U, Schmorl P, Richter-Witte C, Godeke-Koch T, Feutl S, Schramm J, Ludwig H, Johannes S and Emrich HM (2005) Brain potential amplitude varies as a function of Borna disease virus-specific immune complexes in obsessive-compulsive disorder. Molecular Psychiatry 10: 515–515.

Eisen JL, Mancebo MA, Pinto A, Coles ME, Pagano ME, Stout R and Rasmussen SA (2006) Impact of obsessive-compulsive disorder on quality of life. Comprehensive Psychiatry 47: 270–275.

Faith JJ, Guruge JL, Charbonneau M, Subramanian S, Seedorf H and Goodman AL (2013) The long-term stability of the human gut microbiota. Science 341: 1237439.

Griebel G (1995) 5-Hydroxytryptamine-interacting drugs in animal models of anxiety disorders: more than 30 years of research. Pharmacology & Therapeutics 65: 319–395.

Hornig M, Solbrig M, Horscroft N, Weissenbock H and Lipkin WI (2001) Borna disease virus infection of adult and neonatal rats: models for neuropsychiatric disease. The Mechanisms of Neuronal Damage in Virus Infections of the Nervous System. Springer 157–177.

Jiang H, Ling Z, Zhang Y, Mao H, Ma Z, Yin Y, Wang W, Tang W, Tan Z, Shi J, Li L and Raun B (2015) Altered fecal microbiota composition in patients with major depressive disorder. Brain, Behavior, and Immunity 48: 186–194.

Kantak PA, Bobrow DN and Nyby JG (2014) Obsessive–compulsive-like behaviors in house mice are attenuated by a probiotic (Lactobacillus rhamnosus GG). Behavioural Pharmacology 25: 71–79.

Kugler BB, Lewin AB, Phares V, Geffken GR, Murphy TK and Storch EA (2013) Quality of life in obsessive-compulsive disorder: The role of mediating variables. Psychiatry Research 206: 43–49.

Lyte M (2011) Probiotics function mechanistically as delivery vehicles for neuroactive compounds: microbial endocrinology in the design and use of probiotics. Bioessays 33: 574–581.

Maes M, Twisk FN, Kubera M, Ringel K, Leunis JC and Geffard M (2012) Increased IgA responses to the LPS of commensal bacteria is associated with inflammation and activation of cell-mediated immunity in chronic fatigue syndrome. Journal of Affective Disorders 136: 909–917.

Maes M, Ringel K, Kubera M, Anderson G, Morris G, Galecki P and Geffard M (2013) In myalgic encephalomyelitis/chronic fatigue syndrome, increased autoimmune activity against 5-HT is associated with immuno-inflammatory pathways and bacterial translocation. Journal of Affective Disorders 150: 223–230.

Menzies RG and De Silva P (2003) Obsessive-Compulsive Disorder: Theory, Research and Treatment, Chichester, West Sussex, England: Wiley.

Messaoudi M, Lalonde R, Violle N, Javelot H, Desdor D, Nejdi A, Bisson JF, Rougeot C, Pichelin M, Cazaubiel M and Cazaubiel JM (2011a) Assessment of psychotropic-like properties of a probiotic formulation (Lactobacillus helveticus R0052 and Bifidobacterium longum R0175) in rats and human subjects. British Journal of Nutrition 105: 755–764.

Messaoudi M, Violle N, Bisson J-F, Desor D, Javelot H and Rougeot C (2011b) Beneficial psychological effects of a probiotic formulation (Lactobacillus helveticus R0052 and Bifidobacterium longum R0175) in healthy human volunteers. Gut Microbes 2: 256–261.

Miman O, Mutlu EA, Ozcan O, Atambay M, Karlidaq R and Unal S (2010) Is there any role of Toxoplasma gondii in the etiology of obsessive–compulsive disorder? Psychiatry Research 177: 263–265.

Morgan XC, Tickle TL, Sokol H, Gevers D, Devaney KL, Ward DV, Reyes JA, Shah SA, Leleiko N, Snapper SB, Bousvaros A, Korzenik J, Sands BE, Xavier RJ and Huttenhower C (2012) Dysfunction of the intestinal microbiome in inflammatory bowel disease and treatment. Genome Biology 13: 1.

Nadal I, Donant E, Ribes-Koninckx C, Calabuig M and Sanz Y (2007) Imbalance in the composition of the duodenal microbiota of children with coeliac disease. Journal of Medical Microbiology 56: 1669–1674.

Naseribafrouei A, Hestad K, Avershina E, Sekelja M, Linlokken A, Wilson R and Rudi K (2014) Correlation between the human fecal microbiota and depression. Neurogastroenterology and Motility 26: 1155–1162.

Parracho HM, Bingham MO, Gibson GR and McCartney AL (2005) Differences between the gut microflora of children with autistic spectrum disorders and that of healthy children. Journal of Medical Microbiology 54: 987–991.

Pellow S, Johnston AL and File SE (1987) Selective agonists and antagonists for 5-hydroxytryptamine receptor subtypes, and interactions with yohimbine and FG 7142 using the elevated plus-maze test in the rat. Journal of Pharmacy and Pharmacology 39: 917–928.

Qin L, Wu X, Block ML, Liu Y, Breese GR, Hong JS, Knap DJ and Crews FT (2007) Systemic LPS causes chronic neuroinflammation and progressive neurodegeneration. Glia 55: 453–462.

Rees JC (2014) Obsessive–compulsive disorder and gut microbiota dysregulation. Medical Hypotheses 82: 163–166.

Savignac H, Kiely B, Dinan T and Cryan JF (2014) Bifidobacteria exert strain-specific effects on stress-related behavior and physiology in BALB/c mice. Neurogastroenterology and Motility 26: 1615–1627.

Schmidt C (2015) Mental health: thinking from the gut. Nature 518: S12–S15.

Severance EG, Gressitt KL, Stallings CR, Origoni AE, Kushalani S, Leweke FM, Dickerson FB and Yolken RH (2013) Discordant patterns of bacterial translocation markers and implications for innate immune imbalances in schizophrenia. Schizophrenia Research 148: 130–137.

Shanahan NA, Velez LP, Masten VL and Dulawa SC (2011) Essential role for orbitofrontal serotonin 1B receptors in obsessive-compulsive disorder-like behavior and serotonin reuptake inhibitor response in mice. Biological Psychiatry 70: 1039–1048.

Sudo N, Chida Y, Aiba Y, Sonoda J, Oyama N, Yu XN, Kubo C and Koqa Y (2004) Postnatal microbial colonization programs the hypothalamic–pituitary–adrenal system for stress response in mice. The Journal of Physiology 558: 263–275.

Swedo SE (2010) Streptococcal infection, Tourette syndrome, and OCD: is there a connection? PANDAS: horse or zebra? Neurology 74: 1397–1399.

Swedo SE, Seidlitz J, Kovacevic M, Latimer ME, Hommer R, Lougee L and Grant P (2015) Clinical presentation of pediatric autoimmune neuropsychiatric disorders associated with streptococcal infections in research and community settings. Journal of Child and Adolescent Psychopharmacology 25: 26–30.

Turna J, Grosman Kaplan K, Anglin R and Van Ameringen M (2015) What's bugging the gut in OCD? A review of the gut microbiome in obsessive–compulsive disorder. Depression and Anxiety.

Turnbaugh PJ, Ley RE, Mahowald MA, Magrini V, Mardis ER and Gordon JI (2006) An obesity-associated gut microbiome with increased capacity for energy harvest. Nature 444: 1027–1131.

Uher R and McGuffin P (2010) The moderation by the serotonin transporter gene of environmental adversity in the etiology of depression: 2009 update. Molecular Psychiatry 15: 18–22.

Wexler HM (2007) Bacteroides: the good, the bad, and the nitty-gritty. Clinical Microbiology Reviews 20: 593–621.

Zimomra ZR, Porterfield VM, Camp RM and Johnson JD (2011) Time-dependent mediators of HPA axis activation following live *Escherichia coli*. American Journal of Physiology-Regulatory, Integrative and Comparative Physiology 301: R1648–R1657.

Zohar J (2012) Obsessive-compulsive disorder: Current science and clinical practice. Chichester: John Wiley.

Chapter 9

Probiotics and Depression

Derek Larkin[1],* and Colin R Martin[2]

INTRODUCTION

Depression is a common mental disorder, which can be long-lasting or recurrent, substantially impairing an individual's ability to function in their daily life (Vilagut et al., 2016). People with a depressed mood can feel sad, anxious, empty, hopeless, helpless, worthless, guilty, irritable, ashamed or restless (Kim et al., 2015). Individuals may also lose interest in everyday actions such as physical activities, they may lose their appetite or even may find they overeat, many will have difficulties concentrating, or recalling details (Huang et al., 2016). Depressed individuals may also have impairments in decision making, some may even attempt or commit suicide (Kessler et al., 2005). It is widely acknowledged that because of the impact and

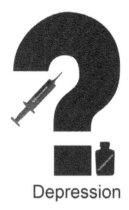

Depression

Figure 1

[1] Edge Hill University, St Helens Road, Ormsirk, Lancashire, L39 4QP.
[2] Faculty of Society and Health, Buckinghamshire New University, Uxbridge Campus, 106 Oxford Road, Uxbridge, Middlesex, UB8 1NA, UK.
* Corresponding author

widespread prevalence, depression is a growing healthcare concern. It is estimated that 1 in 5 of individuals will at some point in their lives, experience depression (Kessler et al., 2005). It is possible that 350 million individuals worldwide currently present with symptoms of depression, but this is likely to be a gross underestimation, and it is thought the problem is steadily increasing (Huang et al., 2016).

Traditionally depression has been treated with a range of therapies including antidepressants and talking therapies, however, research has started to emerge which suggests that probiotics may significantly reduce the symptoms of depression.

Depression

Depression is a multifactorial condition brought about by biological, psychological, and social factors (Naseribafrouei et al., 2014). The diathesis stress model proposes that depression is caused when stressful life events impose on a pre-existing vulnerable condition (Uher and McGuffin, 2010). The handbook of mental disorders, the DSM-5 (APA, 2013), defines depression under the section entitled Depressive Disorders. Depressive disorders include disruptive mood regulation disorder, major depressive disorder, persistent depressive disorder, premenstrual dysphoric disorder, substance/medication-induced depressive disorder, and unspecified depressive disorder. Major depressive disorder represents the classic condition; it is characterized by discrete episodes of at least 2 weeks' duration, although it is acknowledged that in most cases this period is appreciably longer, in which significant changes in affect, cognition, and neurovegetative function and inter-episode remissions are measurably altered (APA, 2013). The shared component of all depressive disorders is the presence of sad, empty, or irritable mood, and the significant loss of the individuals' competency to function. Defining features of all depressive disorders is the duration, timing and etiology (APA, 2013).

Conventional Treatments for Depression

For most individuals diagnosed with a depressive mood disorder the course of treatment will invariably involve a pharmacological antidepressant. The first antidepressants were discovered by accident and were being used as an antitubercular agent, but were found to induce a euphoric effects in patients with tuberculosis (Ramachandraih et al., 2011). This discovery heralded the advent of the antidepressant, and a shift of focus for psychiatrists away from psychodynamic properties of depression, to a biological basis (Ramachandraih et al., 2011). In 1952, Albert Zeller discovered that iproniazid inhibited monoamines oxidase (MOA) enzyme (Maxwell and Eckhardt, 2012). This enzyme causes the oxidation of adrenaline (a monoamine) and is inhibited by ephedrine. MAO enzyme act on a number of endogenous and exogenous amines; serotonin, catecholamines, tyramine, beta-phenylethylamine, and benzylamine. The effects of the administration of iproniazid results in elevated mood, increased appetite (subsequent weight gain), improved sleep, and sociability (Ramachandraih et al., 2011). Early MAO's were not without their side effects such as psychomotor agitation, hyposexuality, and psychoses. The term 'antidepressant' was coined because of the psychostimulatory effects of iproniazid on depressed patients (Ramachandraih et al., 2011). Early data showed that iproniazid significantly improved mood in 70% of patients; the MAO-inhibiting properties of iproniazid increase serotonin secretion in the brain. In spite of the positive results from the administration of iproniazid, it was launched as an antitubercular agent, principally due to hepatic and nephrotoxicity. The early findings did however, lead the way for the development of the first class of exclusive MAO inhibitors such as isocarboxazid, tranylcypromine, phenelzine, mebanazine, nialamide, pheniprazine, and etryptamine (Ramachandraih et al., 2011). Despite the fact that antidepressant medication is widely used to treat depressive symptoms, 30–40% of patients do not respond well to current drug strategies (Rush et al., 2006). Most effective antidepressants potently increase synaptic levels of norepinephrine, and/or serotonin, and in some cases dopamine (Neirenburg et al., 2007). Most antidepressants accomplish this by inhibiting uptake of monoamines noradrenaline, dopamine and serotonin or inhibiting the enzyme MAO. Selective serotonin reuptake inhibitors (SSRI) tend to be the most widely prescribed type of antidepressants. SSRIs tend to increase the extracellular level of the neurotransmitter serotonin by limiting its reabsorption into the presynaptic cell. Serotonin-noradrenaline reuptake inhibitors (SNRI), are thought to work in the same way as SSRI, but with the action of also limiting the reuptake of noradrenaline. Tricyclic antidepressants (TCA) work primarily by increasing levels of norepinephrine and serotonin. In the vast majority of individual's patients treated with antidepressants for depression will see an improvement, however antidepressants tend to come with some serious side-effects. SSRIs and SNRIs, are thought to cause feelings of agitation and anxiety, can make the individual feel sick with digestive and stomach aches often accompanied by diarrhea or constipation. This group of chemicals can also cause dizziness and insomnia headaches and low sex drive. TCAs are thought to cause dry mouth, slight blurring of vision, constipation, problems urinating, drowsiness and weight gain, and changes in heart rhythm. In rare cases individuals taking antidepressants can experience suicidal thoughts and desire to self-harm, a symptom particularly pertinent in people under the age of 25. It is clear therefore antidepressants are extremely useful in the vast majority of cases however they do have many undesired side-effects. Cartwright et al. (2016) found that 30% of individuals in their study reported moderate-to-severe depression on antidepressants. They also found that patients reported sexual problems, and severe weight gain, adverse emotional effects such as feeling emotionally numb.

Probiotics

The World Health Organization (WHO) affirmed that probiotics, as a live microorganism, when taken in prescribed quantities may lead to beneficial health effects of the host (Kennedy et al., 2001). Probiotics are defined as living microorganisms, and was initially used in the 1960s, the word probiotic comes from the Greek word meaning 'for life'. Although the word is relatively new the beneficial effects of certain foods containing live bacteria have been recognized through the centuries (Williams, 2010). The use of probiotics can be traced back to the ancient Greeks and Romans and their use of cheeses and fermented products (Gismondo et al., 1999). In recent years, both research and consumer interest in probiotics has grown. There is an increasing body of clinical evidence that supports the idea that probiotics may have some health benefits, particularly in diarrheal diseases (Williams, 2010). Probiotics are regulated as dietary supplement foods and now are available in capsules, tablets, packets or powders and are contained in various fermented foods most commonly yoghurt or dairy drinks. The probiotic products may contain a single microorganism or mixture of several species (Williams, 2010). The most popular probiotic contains lactic acid bacteria specifically *Lactobacillus* and *Bifidobacterium* species. Specific species of probiotic tend to have particular health benefits, therefore the health benefits attributed to one strain is not necessarily applicable to another, even if the two strains are from the same species (Williams, 2010). The primary rationale for using probiotics involves restoring microbial balance. It is now understood that there are at least 500 different bacterial species living within the adult gastrointestinal tract (Pham et al., 2008). Under normal circumstances a healthy gut flora is generally maintained, however when an individual has undergone surgery or radiation therapy, or is using antibiotics or immunosuppressive medications there may be an increase in pathogenic bacteria which may disrupt the normal gut flora. Under these circumstances the administration of probiotics which contains beneficial bacteria and yeast may restore the microbial balance in the gastrointestinal tract (Santosa et al., 2006). The administration of probiotics may help decrease the number of potentially pathogenic gastrointestinal microorganisms and pathogens and in doing so reduce gastrointestinal discomfort, flatulence, bloating and improved bowel regularity. Probiotics have also been found to enhance the immune response, improve skin function, enhance resistance to certain pollen allergies, and decreased body pathogens as well as protecting DNA, proteins and lipids from oxidative damage (Huang et al., 2016). There is also limited but mounting evidence that probiotics may also have therapeutic effects in relation to liver damage following alcohol abuse (Kirpich et al., 2008).

Recent research appears to show that administration of probiotics may have beneficial health effects beyond the gut. It has been argued that gut probiotics may play a role in bidirectional communication between the gut and the central nervous system (Huang et al., 2016). It has also been proposed that gut microbiota may also have a major influence on an individuals' state of mind (Schmidt, 2015). In recent years there have been several lines of research which have explored gut microbiota in relation to the immune system, brain development and behavior. Gut microbiota has been found to regulate the neurophysiological behaviors through immune, endocrine and neural pathways (Collins et al., 2012). It has also been reported that gut microbiota can be implicated in regulating neurophysiological-governed behaviors, such as stress, autism, pain, and multiple sclerosis (Cryan and Dinan, 2012). It now seems apparent that gut–brain communication is bidirectional (Mu et al., 2016).

Probiotics and Depression

In recent years there has been major interest in exploring the link between the health of the gut and mental health (Schmidt, 2015). Three pathways have been identified that describe how gut microbiota may influence depression, through inflammation, the hypothalamic-pituitary-adrenal axis (HPA), or interference with neurotransmitter signaling (Uher and McGuffin, 2010). Immunoglobulin A (IgA, an antibody that plays a critical role in immune function in the mucous membranes, and the gastrointestinal tract) and immunoglobulin M (IgM, an antibody made in response to infection) mediate inflammation and responses to lipopolysaccharide which have been shown to be elevated in depressed patients (Maes, 2011). A link has also been made that implicates higher inflammatory interleukin 6 (IL-6, an interleukin that acts as both a pro-inflammatory cytokine and an anti-inflammatory myokine) and tumor necrosis factor alpha (TNF-α, involved in systemic inflammation) in depressed patients (Dowlati et al., 2010). Research within an animal model has shown that gastrointestinal inflammation appears to induce anxious behavior, and cause alterations to the central nervous system biochemistry (Bercik et al., 2010).

HPA is a neuro-endocrine response to stress, but also to mood disorders and functional disease (Naseribafrouei et al., 2014). Adjustments to the HPA axis have been observed in individuals with various mental health conditions, including post-traumatic stress disorder, schizophrenia, social anxiety and depression (Naseribafrouei et al., 2014). Research using rats has found that probiotics are able to interfere with the HPA response to acute physiological stress and according to Naseribafrouei et al. (2014) this would indicate a mechanistic connection linking the gut microbiota, HPA and stress.

Direct interference with transmitter signaling may also be linked to depressive states. *Gamma*-Aminobutyric acid (GABA, an inhibitory neurotransmitter) can be produced by intestinal bacteria (Barrett et al., 2012), and probiotics (Bangsgaard Bendtsen et al., 2012) can modify depressive behavior from GABA signaling, at least in the rat model. Other pathways also include serotonergic signaling that has been linked to depression, in which serotonergic turnover is higher in the striatum, again at least in the animal model (Heijtz et al., 2011). Using fecal microbiota as a proxy for gut microbiota, Naseribafrouei et al. (2014) explored the link between fecal microbiota and depressive disorder. They failed to find a direct causal association between intestinal bacteria and depression, they did however find a correlation with low levels of *bacteroidetes* related with depression. Low levels of *bacteroidetes* are normally associated with obesity (Ley et al., 2006). The linkage between adiposity and gut microbial ecology may indicate that manipulation of *bacteroidetes* is more highly associated with obesity than depression. However, the low levels of *bacteroidetes* may also be attributed to low grade inflammation observed in both obesity and depressive disorders (Naseribafrouei et al., 2014). Although the pathways linking gut bacteria with the brain are not fully understood, there is an indication that stress may play a major role (Rook and Lowry, 2008). Fecal microbiome composition in adult rats subjected to maternal separation was dramatically altered in comparison with non-separated controls (O'Mahony et al., 2009) similarly rats subjected to prolonged restraint stressor differed significantly in their microbiota structure compared to non-stressed controls (Bangsgaard Bendtsen et al., 2012). In a study that explored gut microbiota in individuals with major depressive episodes in response to antidepressant treatment Jiang et al. (2015), found differences in gut microbiota associated with major depressive disorder, particularly amongst patients with clinically significant depressive symptoms. This would suggest that intestinal bacteria could possess therapeutic properties for mental illnesses. Desbonnet et al.

(2010) explored the potential benefits of *Bifidobacterium infantis* in rat maternal separation model. They monitored a number of systems including cytokine (immune response markers) that stimulated whole blood samples, monoamine levels in the brain, and peripheral hypothalamic-pituitary-adrenal axis measurements, as well as noradrenaline levels. Rats were subjected to a forced swim test, to assess motivational states. They found that probiotic treatment resulted in normalization of the immune response, a reversal of behavioral deficits and restoration of basal noradrenaline concentrations in the brainstem. This finding appears to show that treatment with a signal bacterium *Bifidobacterium* affects neuronal systems and behaviors relevant to depression in rats exposed to maternal separation stress in early life. These findings appear to indicate the potential benefits of the normalization of intestinal microflora in the regulation of mood and suggest that probiotic bacteria may serve as a therapeutic treatment for depression.

Studies appear to provide evidence which suggest a regulating role for probiotics in relation to the immune response, neuroendocrine, and neurochemical response outside the gastrointestinal tract (Desbonnet et al., 2008; Desbonnet et al., 2010). The lack of probiotic bacteria in the gut may have a detrimental affect not only within the gut, but has been shown to have an adverse effect more centrally within the hypothalamic pituitary adrenal axis and monoaminergic activity, features that have been implicated in the etiology of depression (Desbonnet et al., 2008). The absence of gastrointestinal microbes (in mice) appear to result in reduced expressions of brain derived neurotrophic factor in the cortex, and hippocampus and exaggerated hypothalamic-adrenal-axis response to stress (Sudo et al., 2004). However, the chronic administration of probiotic bacteria (in rats) attenuates the cytokine response to mitogen stimulation and induces an increased peripheral concentration of the serotonin precursor tryptophan, and can have other detrimental effects on various other cortical areas (Desbonnet et al., 2008). But increasing the concentration of specific probiotic *Bifidobacterium* and *Lactobacillus* within the gut appears to increase mood and reduces anxiety symptoms in patients with chronic fatigue syndrome, and irritable bowel syndrome (Desbonnet et al., 2010). In combination, these data appear to suggest that probiotic bacteria positively and negatively influence physical and emotional states.

Stress comes in many forms, and is associated with numerous disorders from depression to irritable bowel syndrome; psychological stress has been shown to alter the composition of intestinal microbiota by decreasing the number of *Bifidobacterium* and *Lactobacillus* (Desbonnet et al., 2010; O'Mahony et al., 2009). The administration of probiotics bacteria appears to attenuate the apparent detrimental effects of stress (Desbonnet et al., 2010). In a double-blind placebo controlled and randomize parallel group study by Messaoudi et al. (2011) rats and healthy human volunteers were administered *Bifidobacterium* and *Lactobacillus* or placebo for 30 days, and were assessed with a battery of psychometric tests, for example, the Hospital Anxiety and Depression Scale (HADS), the Perceived Stress Scale, Urinary Free Cortisol (UFC). Results indicate that daily sub-chronic administration of *Bifidobacterium* and *Lactobacillus* reduced anxiety like behavior in rats, and alleviate psychological distress in human volunteers. In a similar study participants were given a probiotic yoghurt or a multi-species probiotic capsule for six weeks. Mental health parameters including general health questionnaire (GHQ) and depression anxiety and stress scale (DASS) scores were measured. Fasting blood samples were obtained at the beginning and 6 weeks after the intervention to quantify hypothalamic pituitary adrenal axis. Results indicate a significant down regulation in psychological stress levels, and depression scores in participants who regularly took the probiotics (Mohammadi et al., 2015). The frequency of constipation events is significantly correlated with poor mood. In a study that explored the impact on mood related to poor digestive transit and the consumption of a probiotics milk drink, Benton et al. (2007) found that the administration of the probiotic milk drink significantly improve the mood of those previously shown to have low mood, there was however no association found between the frequencies of defecation and improve mood. A study by Akkasheh et al. (2016) examined the effects of probiotics supplementation on symptoms of depression, metabolic profiles serum high sensitivity C reactive protein (hs-CRP) and bio markers of oxidative stress in patients with major depressive disorder (MDD). 40 patients were randomly assigned to either receive probiotic supplementation or a placebo. The probiotic administration was via capsules which contained three viable freeze-dried strains of probiotic: *Lactobacillus acidophilus*, *Lactobacillus casei*, and *Bifidobacterium bifidum*. Following the eight-week intervention patients had significantly decreased their scores on the Beck Depression Inventory (psychometric test for measuring the severity of depression). Evrensel and Ceylan (2015) report that a poor diet has been shown to be a risk factor for depression, as such a healthy diet would to some extent help prevent a depressive state, as such the administration as of probiotics as part of a healthy diet may have critical benefits to the prevention and treatment of depression.

Based on evidence, much of which is presented above, the gut microbiota is strongly implicated with known metabolic disorders such as obesity, diabetes mellitus, and specific neuropsychiatric disorders, which appear to include schizophrenia, autistic spectrum disorder, anxiety disorders and major depressive disorders (Evrensel and Ceylan, 2015).

Psychobiotics

Psychobiotics is an approach that combines two avenues, namely probiotics and psychiatric illness (Dinan et al., 2013). Dinan et al. (2013) describes psychobiotics as "a live organism that, when ingested in adequate amounts, produces a health benefit in patients suffering from psychiatric illness". The National Institute of Health in the USA has funded many projects which appear to be yielding promising results. Currently the Human Microbiome Project is funding projects exploring, pregnancy and preterm birth, onset of inflammatory bowel disease, and onset of Type II diabetes. In 2012 Thomas Insel, Director of the National Institute of Mental Health in the USA, referred to the study of macrobiotics "How these differences in our microbial would influence the development of the brain and behavior will be one of the greatest frontiers of clinical neuroscience in the next decade" (Insel, 2012). Research in recent years appears to be yielding promising results which indicate that cognitive and emotional processes can be altered by microbes acting through the brain–gut axis (Dinan et al., 2013; Heijtz et al., 2011).

Discussion

The prevalence of individuals affected by mental health disorders has been the focus of significant interest over recent decades. What is clear is the rate of diagnosis has increased substantially and a growing number of children and adolescents are now requiring pharmacological and psychotherapy treatments as well as educational interventions (Polanczyk et al., 2015). There is however, evidence to suggest that on occasions individuals are over diagnosed and over treated (James et al., 2014). Depression is a complex and multifactorial disorder involving marked disabilities in global functioning with multiple comorbidities. Over the last few decades' anti-depressants have been developed that are, on the whole, well-tolerated, and target serotonin, and/or norepinephrine, primarily. However, not all patients respond well to pharmacological interventions. Some of the side effects can almost be far more detrimental than the underlying condition.

Probiotics are proposed to have a range of health benefits, the benefits are thought to include relief from irritable bowel syndrome, Inflammatory bowel disease and may even help in the prevention of bowel cancer (Akkasheh et al., 2016). There is an increasing body of research which has reported that the microflora of the intestines may affect the immune system and function beyond the gut. And it is clear from research that probiotics might have favorable effects on mood and psychological problems. Applications of particular probiotics appear to reverse the behavioral effects of depression and normalize immune response and doing so normalize basal intestinal microbiota, a positive therapeutic application that is to a large extent being ignored or overlooked.

In spite of the promises made by Thomas Insel, Director of the National Institute of Mental Health in the USA, an in-depth analysis of microbiota in depression and other stress-related disorders has not fulfilled its early potential. However preclinical data strongly supports the view that an aberrant microbiota may alter behavior, immunity, and endocrinology (Dinan et al., 2013). The aberrant microbiota may however be replaced with healthy flora by the administration of healthy gut bacteria.

References

Akkasheh G, Kashani-Poor Z, Tajabadi-Ebrahimi M, Jafari P, Akbari H, Taghizadeh M, Memarzadeh MR, Asemi Z and Esmaillzadeh A (2016) Clinical and metabolic response to probiotic administration in patients with major depressive disorder: A randomized, double-blind, placebo-controlled trial. Nutrition 32(3): 315–320. doi:10.1016/j.nut.2015.09.003.

APA (2013) Diagnostic and Statistical Manual of Mental Disorders 5th Edition. Washington, DC: American Psychiatric Association.

Bangsgaard Bendtsen KM, Krych L, Sørensen DB, Pang W, Nielsen DS, Josefsen K, Hansen LH, Sørensen SJ and Hansen AK (2012) Gut microbiota composition is correlated to grid floor induced stress and behavior in the BALB/c mouse. PloS One 7(10): e46231. doi:10.1371/journal.pone.0046231.

Barrett E, Ross R, O'Toole P, Fitzgerald G and Stanton C (2012) γ-Aminobutyric acid production by culturable bacteria from the human intestine. Journal of Applied Microbiology 113(2): 411–417. doi:10.1111/j.1365-2672.2012.05344.x.

Benton D, Williams C and Brown A (2007) Impact of consuming a milk drink containing a probiotic on mood and cognition. European Journal of Clinical Nutrition 61(3): 355–361. doi:10.1038/sj.ejcn.1602546.

Bercik P, Verdu EF, Foster JA, Macri J, Potter M, Huang X, Malinowski P, Jackson W, Blennerhassett P, Neufeld KA, Lu J, Khan WI, Corthesy-Theulaz I, Cherbut C, Bergonzelli GE and Collins SM

(2010) Chronic gastrointestinal inflammation induces anxiety-like behavior and alters central nervous system biochemistry in mice. Gastroenterology 139(6): 2102–2112.e2101. doi:10.1053/j. gastro.2010.06.063.

Cartwright C, Gibson K, Read J, Cowan O and Dehar T (2016) Long-term antidepressant use: patient perspectives of benefits and adverse effects. Patient Preference and Adherence 10: 1401–1407. doi:10.2147/PPA.S110632.

Collins SM, Surette M and Bercik P (2012) The interplay between the intestinal microbiota and the brain. Nat Rev Micro 10(11): 735–742. doi:10.1038/nrmicro2876.

Cryan JF and Dinan TG (2012) Mind-altering microorganisms: the impact of the gut microbiota on brain and behaviour. Nature Reviews Neuroscience 13(10): 701–712. doi:10.1038/nrn3346.

Desbonnet L, Garrett L, Clarke G, Bienenstock J and Dinan T (2008) The probiotic Bifidobacteria infantis: An assessment of potential antidepressant properties in the rat. Journal of Psychiatric Research 43(2): 164–174. doi:10.1016/j.jpsychires.2008.03.009.

Desbonnet L, Garrett L, Clarke G, Kiely B, Cryan JF and Dinan TG (2010) Effects of the probiotic Bifidobacterium infantis in the maternal separation model of depression. Neuroscience 170(4): 1179–1188. doi:10.1016/j.neuroscience.2010.08.005.

Dinan TG, Stanton C and Cryan JF (2013) Psychobiotics: A novel class of psychotropic. Biological Psychiatry 74(10): 720–726. doi:10.1016/j.biopsych.2013.05.001.

Dowlati Y, Herrmann N, Swardfager W, Liu H, Sham L, Reim EK and Lanctôt KL (2010) A meta-analysis of cytokines in major depression. Biological Psychiatry 67(5): 446–457. doi:10.1016/j. biopsych.2009.09.033.

Evrensel A and Ceylan ME (2015) The gut–brain axis: The missing link in depression. Clinical Psychopharmacology and Neuroscience 13(3): 239–244. doi:10.9758/cpn.2015.13.3.239.

Gismondo MR, Drago L and Lombardi A (1999) Review of probiotics available to modify gastrointestinal flora. International Journal of Antimicrobial Agents 12(4): 287–292. doi:10.1016/S0924-8579(99)00050-3.

Heijtz RD, Wang S, Anuar F, Qian Y, Björkholm B, Samuelsson A, Hibberd ML, Forssberg H and Pettersson S (2011) Normal gut microbiota modulates brain development and behavior. Proceedings of the National Academy of Sciences 108(7): 3047–3052. doi:10.1073/pnas.1010529108.

Huang R, Wang K and Hu J (2016) Effect of Probiotics on Depression: A systematic review and meta-analysis of randomized controlled trials. Nutrients 8(8): 483. doi:10.3390/nu8080483.

Insel T (2012) National Institute of Mental Health. Director's Blog. Retrieved from http://www.nimh.nih. gov/about/director/index.shtml.

James A, Hoang U, Seagroatt V, Clacey J, Goldacre M and Leibenluft E (2014) A comparison of American and English hospital discharge rates for pediatric bipolar disorder, 2000 to 2010. Journal of the American Academy of Child and Adolescent Psychiatry 53(6): 614–624. doi:10.1016/j. jaac.2014.02.008.

Jiang H, Ling Z, Zhang Y, Mao H, Ma Z, Yin Y, Wang W, Tan Z, Shi J, Li L and Ruan B (2015) Altered fecal microbiota composition in patients with major depressive disorder. Brain, Behavior, and Immunity 48: 186–194. doi:10.1016/j.bbi.2015.03.016.

Kennedy R, Kirk S and Gardiner K (2001) Probiotics (Br J Surg 2001; 88: 161–2). The British Journal of Surgery 88(7): 1018. doi:10.1046/j.1365-2168.2001.01850-12.x.

Kessler RC, Berglund P, Demler O, Jin R, Merikangas KR and Walters EE (2005) Lifetime prevalence and age-of-onset distributions of DSM-IV disorders in the national comorbidity survey replication. Archives of General Psychiatry 62(6): 593–602. doi:10.1001/archpsyc.62.6.593.

Kim JL, Cho J, Park S and Park E-C (2015) Depression symptom and professional mental health service use. BMC Psychiatry 15(1): 261. doi:10.1186/s12888-015-0646-z.

Kirpich I, Solovieva N, Leikhter S, Shidakova N, Lebedeva O, Sidorov P, Bazhukova T, Soloviev AG, Barve SS, McClain CJ and Cave M (2008) Probiotics restore bowel flora and improve liver enzymes in human alcohol-induced liver injury: A pilot study. Alcohol 42(8): 675–682. doi:doi:10.1016/j. alcohol.2008.08.006.

Ley RE, Turnbaugh PJ, Klein S and Gordon JI (2006) Microbial ecology: human gut microbes associated with obesity. Nature 444(7122): 1022–1023. doi:10.1038/4441022a.

Maes M (2011) An intriguing and hitherto unexplained co-occurrence: Depression and chronic fatigue syndrome are manifestations of shared inflammatory, oxidative and nitrosative (IO&NS) pathways. Progress in Neuro-Psychopharmacology and Biological Psychiatry 35(3): 784–794. doi:10.1016/j.pnpbp.2010.06.023.

Maxwell RA and Eckhardt SB (2012) Drug discovery: a casebook and analysis. Springer Science & Business Media.

Messaoudi M, Lalonde R, Violle N, Javelot H, Desor D, Nejdi A, Bisson JF, Rougeot C, Pichelin M, Cazaubiel M and Cazaubiel JM (2011) Assessment of psychotropic-like properties of a probiotic formulation (Lactobacillus helveticus R0052 and Bifidobacterium longum R0175) in rats and human subjects. British Journal of Nutrition 105(05): 755–764. doi:10.1017/S0007114510004319.

Mohammadi AA, Jazayeri S, Khosravi-Darani K, Solati Z, Mohammadpour N, Asemi Z, Adab Z, Djalali M, Tehrani-Doost M, Hosseini M and Eghtesadi S (2015) The effects of probiotics on mental health and hypothalamic–pituitary–adrenal axis: A randomized, double-blind, placebo-controlled trial in petrochemical workers. Nutritional Neuroscience.

Mu C, Yang Y and Zhu W (2016) Gut Microbiota: The brain peacekeeper. Frontiers in Microbiology 7: 345. doi:10.3389/fmicb.2016.00345.

Naseribafrouei A, Hestad K, Avershina E, Sekelja M, Linløkken A, Wilson R and Rudi K (2014) Correlation between the human fecal microbiota and depression. Neurogastroenterology and Motility 26(8): 1155–1162. doi:10.1111/nmo.12378.

Neirenburg A, Ostacher M, Delgado P, Sachs G, Gelenberg A, Rosenbaum J and Fava M (2007) Antidepressants and anti-manic medication. In: Gabbard GO (Ed.). Gabbard's Treatments of Psychiatric Disorders (4th ed.). American Psychiatric Publishing Inc.

O'Mahony SM, Marchesi JR, Scully P, Codling C, Ceolho AM, Quigley EMM, Cryan JF and Dinan TG (2009) Early life stress alters behavior, immunity, and microbiota in rats: Implications for irritable bowel syndrome and psychiatric illnesses. Biological Psychiatry 65(3): 263–267. doi:10.1016/j.biopsych.2008.06.026.

Pham M, Lemberg DA and Day AS (2008) Probiotics: sorting the evidence from the myths. Medical Journal of Australia 189(3): 182–182.

Polanczyk GV, Salum GA, Sugaya LS, Caye A and Rohde LA (2015) Annual research review: A meta-analysis of the worldwide prevalence of mental disorders in children and adolescents. Journal of Child Psychology and Psychiatry 56(3): 345–365. doi:10.1111/jcpp.12381.

Ramachandraih CT, Subramanyam N, Bar KJ, Baker G and Yeragani VK (2011) Antidepressants: From MAOIs to SSRIs and more. Indian Journal of Psychiatry 53(2): 180–182. doi:10.4103/0019-5545.82567.

Rook GAW and Lowry CA (2008) The hygiene hypothesis and psychiatric disorders. Trends in Immunology 29(4): 150–158. doi:10.1016/j.it.2008.01.002.

Rush J, Trivedi M, Wisniewski S, Nierenberg AA, Stewart J, Warden D, Niederehe G, Thase ME, Lavori PW, Lebowitz BD, McGrath PJ, Rosenbaum JF, Sackeim HA, Kupfer DJ, Luther J and Fava M (2006) Acute and longer-term outcomes in depressed outpatients requiring one or several treatment steps: A STAR*D report. American Journal of Psychiatry 163(11): 1905–1917. doi:10.1176/ajp.2006.163.11.1905.

Santosa S, Farnworth E and Jones PJ (2006) Probiotics and their potential health claims. Nutrition Reviews 64(6): 265–274. doi:10.1111/j.1753-4887.2006.tb00209.x.

Schmidt C (2015) Mental health: thinking from the gut. Nature 518(7540): S12–S15. doi:10.1038/518S13a.

Sudo N, Chida Y, Aiba Y, Sonoda J, Oyama N, Yu XN and Koga Y (2004) Postnatal microbial colonization programs the hypothalamic–pituitary–adrenal system for stress response in mice. The Journal of Physiology 558(1): 263–275. doi:10.1113/jphysiol.2004.063388.

Uher R and McGuffin P (2010) The moderation by the serotonin transporter gene of environmental adversity in the etiology of depression: 2009 update. Molecular Psychiatry 15(1): 18–22. doi:10.1038/mp.2009.123.

Vilagut G, Forero CG, Barbaglia G and Alonso J (2016) Screening for depression in the general population with the Center for Epidemiologic Studies Depression (CES-D): A systematic review with meta-analysis. PloS One 11(5): e0155431.

Williams NT (2010) Probiotics. American Journal of Health-System Pharmacy 67(6): 449–458. doi:10.2146/ajhp090168.

Chapter 10

Probiotics and Alcohol Dependency

Derek Larkin[1],* and Colin R Martin[2]

INTRODUCTION

The effects of chronic alcohol dependency are well documented, and can range from social dysfunction to serious medical complications. Less well documented are the therapeutic roles of probiotics in relation to chronic alcohol consumption, particularly in regard to alcohol-induced liver disease and bowel flora.

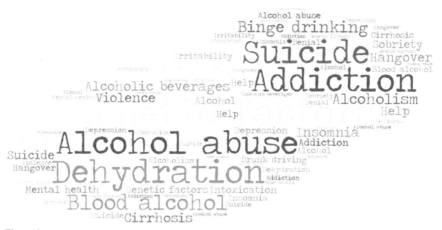

Figure 1

---

[1] Edge Hill University, St Helens Road, Ormsirk, Lancashire, L39 4QP.
[2] Faculty of Society and Health, Buckinghamshire New University, Uxbridge Campus, 106 Oxford Road, Uxbridge, Middlesex, UB8 1NA, UK.
* Corresponding author

Long before the invention of the microscope, theories were abound concerning tiny creatures, invisible to the naked eye, which caused diseases by entering the body through the mouth and nose. Even so, in more recent history such theories were discounted, and most dismissed the idea that organisms like bacteria and germs could cause illnesses. Disease and ill health were thought of as spontaneous occupancies, even the father of microbiology, Antonie van Leeuwenhoek, could not reconcile the creatures he saw under his microscope and the idea that they could cause diseases.

It took a long time but eventually, with greater scientific methods and close observation, it was acknowledged that bacteria could cause disease. It is now general knowledge that some bacteria can cause ill health in human and other animals, while other are either harmless or even beneficial. The beneficial bacteria are what we now call probiotics.

Probiotics (from Pro thought to be from the Latin meaning 'for' and Biotics thought to be from the Greek meaning 'Life') are described as live microbial feed supplements, which beneficially affect the host animal by improving its intestinal microbial balance (Fuller, 1989). Probiotics are thought to have a beneficial effect on the host by increasing its intestinal microbial population, which is thought to help inhibit pathogens. Our intestinal system is home to some 500 different forms of bacteria, which live in a symbiotic fashion with our gut, helping to keep us healthy and assist in the digestion of food. Probiotics can be taken as a supplement in the form of live yoghurt and some foods have probiotic properties such as Kifer (a cross between yoghurt and milk) dark chocolate, and some soft cheeses, among others. Some products however, have probiotics added to them to help infer a healthy aura, but some products such as milk with added probiotics are not recommended to the very young or the very old because of the risk of excess gas or stomach bloating. Probiotics are after all live bacteria, and introducing live cultures into an already compromised or weakened immune system can be potentially very harmful. So even though probiotics may mean 'pro-life' probiotics may not be beneficial for everyone, particularly those with a compromised immune system.

When we drink alcohol about 20% is absorb by the stomach, the other 80% is absorbed by the small intestine. The rate at which alcohol is absorb is dependent on several factors, for example, a full stomach will slow down the absorption of alcohol; the type of drink containing alcohol is also a factor, spirits will be absorbed much faster than beer, or wine, because of the concentration of alcohol in the liquid.

Once the alcohol enters the blood stream the body is simultaneously attempting to absorb and trying to remove it. Several systems come into play; the kidneys and the lungs remove about 10% and the liver breaks down the rest into acetic acid. Alcohol is toxic and there aren't many bodily systems that are not affected by its consumption. Most adults will have learnt first-hand of its influence on our mood, on our ability to perform well-practiced tasks like walking, talking or driving. In high enough quantities, we can go from feelings of euphoria, excitement, confusion, stupor, to coma and even death. Death can be a slow chronic condition, which we'll talk about next, or it can be relatively fast, when the blood alcohol concentration reaches 0.50% the person's heart may slow, breathing may become laboured and shallow, and even stop, leading to death. In much smaller concentrations, the effect of alcohol can be felt on the biochemistry of the brain. Alcohol influences the way the brain send signals the others bodily systems, by altering the levels of neurotransmitters. Neurotransmitters are chemical messengers that allow neurones to send signals to other neurones or glands, which control our behaviour, movement, every thought and feeling. The biochemistry of the brain is a complex symphony of activity, which can be easily disordered and disturbed by alcohol. Long-term dependency on alcohol can lead to permanent damage, which can lead to brain atrophy (cell death). Long-term dependency on alcohol can also lead to a condition called Wernicke-Korsakoff syndrome; in this chronic condition the body fails to absorb thiamine (a B vitamin). Thiamine is used in the biosynthesis of several neurotransmitters.

The stomach also suffers damage through the long-term use of alcohol principally because alcohol irritates the stomach lining, which can cause long-term damage, even stomach ulcers. Within the first phase of digestion a complex symphony of chemical processes takes place, which readies the body for consumption of food and fluids. When food first enters the mouth, saliva immediately starts to breakdown the meal, with help from the grinding action of the teeth. The mouth is also home to many bacteria (mostly harmless), most of which will be killed by acids in the stomach, others however may stay in the mouth and cause tooth or gum decay. Once swallowed food follows the path of the digestive system also known as the gastrointestinal tract (GI)—mouth-throat-esophagus-stomach-small intestine-and large intestine. In essence, the GI performs two vital functions, the breaking down and absorption of nutrients, alongside the prevention of absorption of harmful substances such as alcohol. An action called peristalsis transports food around the GI—muscles contract in a wave like action so food is gently conveyed from one vital region to the next.

Other systems such as the liver and gut are also particularly sensitive to alcohol consumption as these are the organs that help breakdown alcohol into smaller less harmful substances for removal from the body. Alcohol has no nutritional value whatsoever, and we can happily live without ever needing to take an alcoholic beverage. The toxic effects of alcohol are however far reaching. Long-term alcohol use can lead to alcoholic hepatitis (inflammation of the liver)—with symptoms that include nausea, vomiting, fever, loss of appetite, and most people with this condition go on to develop cirrhosis, which means the liver becomes unable to function because of scar tissue.

Under normal circumstances most individuals will not reach the stage of liver damage after just a few glasses of wine or drinking heavily during a Stag or Hen do, the human body is very resilient to these rare events. But some people have long-term problems with alcohol. The American Medical Association (AMA) defines alcoholism or alcohol dependence as "a primary, chronic disease with genetic, psychosocial, and environmental factors influencing its development and manifestations". The NHS in the UK estimates that 9% of men and 4% of women show signs of alcohol dependency. When an individual is dependent on alcohol, they're at an increased risk of developing high blood pressure, stroke, coronary heart disease and liver disease. Prolonged heavy drinking damages the liver. An estimated seven out of 10 people with alcoholic liver disease have an alcohol dependency problem. The most serious form of alcoholic liver disease—cirrhosis, means the liver has been scarred from continuous, long-term damage. Scar tissue replaces healthy tissue in the liver and prevents the liver from working properly. If the individual develops cirrhosis, cutting out alcohol completely is essential to prevent death from liver failure. In the most serious cases of cirrhosis, it is the effect on the liver that has gained most attention in regard to the beneficial effects of pre- and pro-biotics.

In liver health, the main effect of probiotics might occur through the prevention or uptake of lipopolysaccharides, which are found in the outer portion of the gram-negative bacteria, which act as endotoxins and can elicit a strong immune response (Gratz et al., 2010).

There is a close relationship between the liver and the gut; blood from the intestine and gut activates liver-functions (Cesaro et al., 2011), and in a reciprocal manner the liver activates intestinal functions through the secretion of bile into the intestinal lumen. The intestinal microbiota form a complex ecological system, which participates in the production of vitamins, degradation of bile acids, the digestions of nutrients and performs a vital role in immunity. Alongside these roles the intestinal mucosa (comprising of epithelium, lamina propria, and lamina muscularis mucosae), the endogenous intestinal flora form an important barrier against pathogens (Cesaro et al., 2011).

There are numerous ways to cause insult on the liver (be it, viral, toxic or metabolic) the onset of inflammation, steatosis, fibrosis or cirrhosis, share this common path, alterations to the intestinal microbiota appear to perform a vital role in the induction and progression of liver damage. Probiotics however, may mitigate some of the pathogenic alterations in the generation and advancement of chronic liver disease.

Research encompassing the beneficial role of probiotics in alcohol dependency is at the moment limited, most of the research has concentrated on the effects of probiotics and liver health and liver damage following alcohol abuse. Kirpich et al. (2008) conducted a pilot study in which they examined 66 males, hospitalised for reasons of alcohol abuse, and had been diagnosed with alcoholic psychosis, a condition in which patients suffers from delusions and hallucinations. The male patients were randomly assigned to experimental condition 1, in which they were given 5 days of Bifidobacterium bifidum and Lactobacillus plantarum 8PA3 plus absence from alcohol, experimental condition 2 amounted to 5 days of abstinence from alcohol and vitamin supplements. Data from these conditions were compared with 24 match controls that had not consumed alcohol. The results indicate that the probiotic group (experimental condition) demonstrated specific alterations in the bowel flora. The previously depressed numbers of bifidobacteria, lactobacilli, and enterococci, in the experimental group, had returned to numbers seen in healthy controls. Before the study began the experimenters explored liver function and found that aspartate aminotransferase (AST), alanine aminotransferase (ALT) and Gamma-glutamyltransferase (GGT) liver enzymes were significantly elevated. However, after treatment the enzyme levels had improved. Nevertheless, the enzyme AST was the only enzyme that reached statistically significant improvement. This enzyme however is not specifically related to liver damage; it could have been elevated before the experiment trials as a result of other tissue damage. The enzyme ALT is however associated with liver damage and was found to be elevated before the experiment trial, but was found to be much improved after the probiotic treatment.

The present study demonstrates several potentially important and novel results. First, it was the largest study to date demonstrating specific alterations in the bowel flora of alcoholics. Secondly, this was the first human pilot study demonstrating a potential therapeutic role for probiotics in the short-term treatment of ALD. Probiotic therapy was associated with an increase in the number of faecal bifidobacteria and lactobacilli. This suggests that probiotic therapy played a causal role in the improvement in liver enzymes (Kirpich et al., 2008).

This all seems positive, but there are several critical points that need to be made, these points don't necessarily weaken the results but they do need addressing nevertheless. Under ideal circumstances a clinical study would involve a double-blind methodology, using this technique neither the technician administering the drug/treatment or the patient would know whether the patient is in an experimental group or a placebo group. In the present study involved open label methodology in which the patient and the administrating technician were not blinded to the group assignment. And of course, there was no placebo group, therefore, any change in bowel flora or liver enzyme may have been due to chance or act of will. Not to distract from the overarching findings there does seem to be some beneficial effects in the probiotic therapy group. However, it is difficult to tribute cause and effect without a true clinical double-blind study.

A study conducted at University College London, assigned patients with alcoholic cirrhosis, to two groups (Stadlbauer et al., 2008). Twelve were assigned a treatment of Lactobacillus casei shirota supplements (a bacterium generally found in the mouth and intestines; this strain has been shown to be particularly beneficial in inhibiting the growth of Helicobacter pylori, a bacterium linked to the development of duodenal ulcers and stomach cancer, but only disappointingly *in vivo*). The other 8 patients were assigned to the control group, alongside 13 healthy volunteers who received no probiotics. Again, this is a very small study, with no placebo group, and was again not double blinded. Therefore, the experimental group were fully aware of receiving the probiotic treatment/supplement, and just as importantly the control groups were aware of no treatment plan. Nevertheless, the authors maintain that changes in the experimental group were significant. They report the before the introduction of probiotics those with alcoholic cirrhosis had a compromised neutrophil phagocyte capacity, whereas after the treatment this capacity had stabilized in the experimental group, but there was no change in the alcohol cirrhosis controls.

Individuals who have alcoholic cirrhosis generally have a much-compromised immune response, leaving them susceptible to infections. The authors of this paper suggest that their research adds to the increasing body of evidence indicating that treatment of friendly bacteria may boost the immune system in alcoholics.

This would seem very powerful evidence in favour of the beneficial aspects of probiotic supplements; however, there is another word of caution that needs to be expressed, a major probiotics manufacturer helped sponsor this research. This does not fully negate the findings, but a critical approach must be exercised, simply because if there had been no beneficial effect of the probiotic would the research had been published, probably not.

References

Cesaro C, Tiso A, Del Prete A, Cariello R, Tuccillo C, Cotticelli G and DelVecchio Blanco C (2011) Gut microbiota and probiotics in chronic liver diseases. Digestive Liver Disease 43: 431–438.

Fuller R (1989) Probiotics in man and animals. The Journal of Applied Bacteriology 66: 365–378.

Gratz S, Mykkanen H and El-Nezami HS (2010) Probiotic and gut health: a special focus on liver diseases. World Journal of Gastroenterology 28: 403–410.

Kirpich I, Solovieva N, Leikhter S, Shidakova NA, Lebedeva OV, Sidorov PI, Bazhukova TA, Soloviev AG, Barves SS, McClain CJ and Cave M (2008) Probiotics restore bowel flora and improve liver enzymes in human alcohol-induced liver injury: A pilot study. Alcohol 42: 675–682.

Stadlbauer V, Mookerjee R, Hodges S, Wright GA, Davies NA and Jalan R (2008) Effect of probiotic treatment on deranged neutrophil function and cytokine responses in patients with compensated alcoholic cirrhosis. Journal of Hepatology 48: 945–951.

CHAPTER 11

Probiotics and their Potential Effects on Schizophrenia Symptoms

Mick P Fleming[1],* and Colin R Martin[2]

INTRODUCTION

Schizophrenia is a complex multi-factorial mental health problem characterised by severe and intrusive psychic symptoms and debilitating social and emotional symptoms. The conceptual framework for the syndrome of schizophrenia has its historical roots in Kraepelins decade long observation of the onset, course and outcome of mental disorders (Kraepelin, 1913). Initially envisaged as a degenerative condition predominantly effecting young males, Kraepelin applied the term 'dementia praecox'. The onset was in late teens or adolescence and the course was one of gradual deterioration to an end state where the outcome was described with the use of terms such as idiocy, psychological weakness, feeble-minded confusion and cognitive disorganisation (Kraepelin, 1913). Bleuler (1911) applied the term schizophrenia to dementia praecox because he disagreed that the course of the disorder did not always end in intellectual deterioration (dementia), could occur in middle or later life and did not always occur in late teens (praecox). Consequently, he thought this made the term dementia praecox redundant (Bentall, 2009). He applied the term schizophrenia because the term refers to 'schiz' or a splitting and 'phren' meaning mind. Bleuler (1911) thought that this described the process of splitting of the various mental functions from each other. In his view, this disintegration or disconnection in psychic functioning led to the development of symptoms such as hallucinations and delusions (Clare, 1976; Bentall, 2009).

[1] Senior Lecturer, Learning Education and Development (LEaD), Cabinet Office, Isle of Man Government.
[2] Professor of Mental Health, Faculty of Society and Health, New Buckinghamshire University.
* Corresponding author

The schizophrenia syndrome is characterised by severe thought disorder and disturbances to perception. The diagnostic criterion for schizophrenia is written into diagnostic manuals ICD10/DSMIV (WHO, 1992; APA, 1994). A diagnosis of schizophrenia is based on the presence of at least two symptoms which persist for a time period of at least one to six months. The symptoms that characterise schizophrenia are positive symptoms, those behaviours and experiences that would preferably be absent such as hallucinations in any of the five modalities (auditory, visual, olfactory, touch, taste), delusions, disorders of stream and content of thought, and negative symptoms. The second category of symptoms is based on the absence of desired behaviours and the terms used to describe these symptoms are deficit syndrome or more commonly negative symptoms. Based on the finding that distinct neuroanatomical differences were found in people that presented with negative symptoms compared to people that did not present with those symptoms (Crow, 1980). The presentation of negative symptoms is characterised by a lack of enjoyment, cognitive impairment, a lack of motivation, emotional flatness and poverty of thought and speech (Crow, 1980; Andreason, 1982). Such presentations have been viewed as progressive, to have a poor prognosis and are generally irreversible (Crow, 1985).

The average of onset of schizophrenia for women has been found to be 25–30 years (Goldstein and Kreisma, 1988; Raji et al., 2009) compared to a range of 18–25 years for men (Goldstein and Lewine, 2000; Raji et al., 2009). A combination of treatment effects, the debilitating effects of the symptoms, stigma and the effects of social exclusion can result in severe impairments of physical, social, emotional and life functioning in people that have schizophrenia (Martin and Fleming, 2009). The average annual incidence of schizophrenia has been found to range from 15 per 100,000 persons to 40 per 100,000, the average figures for prevalence are approximately 4.5 per 1,000 persons and the risk of developing the illness over a person's lifetime is 0.7% (Tandon et al., 2008). Bentall (2009) made the calculation that some form of psychoses affects 200 million people worldwide. Studies have found that a third of people diagnosed with schizophrenia make a full recovery, another third will show a gradual improvement but will not fully recover to pre-morbid functioning, and a third will remain ill with continued need for hospitalisation (Harding et al., 1987).

Despite criticisms over the lack of homogenous characteristics within this conceptual model of schizophrenia it has become a universal framework providing consistent diagnostic and treatment responses across many countries and cultures. This concept of schizophrenia is the dominant framework of symptom/experience categories or outcomes for clinical treatments, research, evaluation and other trials (Kendell and Jablensky, 2003).

Probiotics

Probiotics are live bacteria based microorganisms that are non-pathogenic in their nature and when taken in sufficient amount influence the flora in the gut to produce health and immunological improvements (WHO, 2002; Reid et al., 2003; Santosa et al., 2006). A large amount and variety of micro flora and bacteria dwell and colonise within the gastrointestinal tract primarily in the colon. A homeostasis exists between the pathogenic and beneficial bacteria that exist in the gastrointestinal tract. This balance plays a crucial role in supporting a healthy immune system. This is achieved by protecting the body from infection by facilitating the extraction of vitamins and nutrients from digested food. Healthy bacteria compete with unhealthy bacteria for the available vitamins and nutrients helping to maintain the homeostasis within the gastro intestinal tract. This balance can be upset by the introduction of large amounts of pathogenic bacteria or through forms of medical treatment such as the taking of anti-biotics. The continuous introduction of safe and robust probiotics in the form of yeast or bacteria in sufficient amounts that can attach to the intestinal epithelium can stabilise the balance of pathogenic and beneficial bacteria, ensuring support for the immune system (Toedter-Williams, 2010). The benefits of probiotics are strain specific with each specific strain having its own action and providing different benefits for the host (Weichselbaum, 2010). As well as influencing intestinal pH and introducing nutrition for the coloncytes, probiotics further support the immune system by positively affecting immunological production, antibody and cellular immune response (Santosa et al., 2006).

Probiotics and Schizophrenia Symptoms

There is very limited literature which explores direct relationships between probiotics and the symptoms of schizophrenia. An initial literature search identified only one paper that investigated the effect of probiotics directly on the symptoms of schizophrenia (details of search terms and search limiters are provided in Figure 1). This study explored the effect of probiotic treatment on the negative symptoms of schizophrenia in a single male patient (Nagamine et al., 2012).

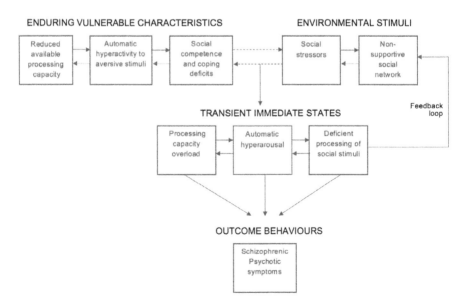

Figure 1 Stress Vulnerability Model (Nuchterlein and Dawson, 1984a).

Table 1 Details of literature search strategy.

Search terms	Search options	Databases	Results
Schizophrenia AND Probiotics	Limiters—Full Text Search Modes Boolean/Phrase	Interface-EBSCOhost Search screen—Advanced search Database—eBook Collection (EBSCOhost); CINAHL, Plus with Full Text; Health Source: Nursing/Academic Edition; MEDLINE; PsycBOOKS; PsycINFO; SocINDEX with Full Text	1

In a single case study design, Nagamine et al. (2012) found that treatment with probiotics had an effect on the alleviation of negative symptoms, in a 50-year-old hospitalised male patient with a 30-year history of schizophrenia, compared to a similar control patient. The man's presentation included both positive (auditory hallucinations) and negative (inactivity, lacking vigour and poor emotional expression) symptoms. The man had also been experiencing chronic constipation and in order to alleviate the constipation a probiotic treatment was administered. The probiotic treatment was composed of three grammes of Streptococcus faecalis per day, Clostridium butyricum and Bacillus mesentericus. The probiotic preparation was made up of 30 milligrammes of Lactomin (S. faecalis), 150 milligrammes of Clostridium butyricum and 150 milligrammes of Bacillus mesentericus. This preparation was administered along with the patient's normal antipsychotic medication regime (haloperidol 1260 milligrammes chlorpromazine equivalent per day and three milligrammes per day biperiden for the relief of extrapyramidal symptoms). The patient acting as control was of a similar age from the same clinical area. This patient was given his usual antipsychotic treatment (haloperidol 1100 milligrammes chlorpromazine equivalent per day and three milligrammes per day biperiden for the relief of extrapyramidal symptoms).

Outcomes were measured using the Positive and Negative Syndrome Scale (PANSS) (Kay et al., 1989). The PANSS is a 30-item gold standard severity measure of the positive and negative symptoms of schizophrenia with a third sub-scale measuring general psychopathology. It is made up of seven items measuring the positive symptoms (delusions, conceptual disorganisation, hallucinatory behaviour, excitement, grandiosity, suspiciousness/persecution and hostility) and seven items measuring the negative symptoms (blunted affect, emotional withdrawal, poor rapport, passive/apathetic social withdrawal, difficulty in abstract thinking, lack of spontaneity and flow of conversation and stereotyped thinking). The remaining 16 items make up the general psychopathology sub-scale (somatic concerns, anxiety, guilt feelings, tension, mannerisms and posturing, depression, motor retardation, uncooperativeness, unusual thought content, disorientation, poor attention, lack of judgment and insight, disturbance of volition, poor impulse control preoccupation and active social avoidance). Each item is scored on a numerical 1–7 likert severity rating from absent (score 1) through to extreme (score 7) giving a scoring range of 30–210, higher scores indicating more serious presentations (Kay et al., 2006). The PANSS is administered through a 30–40 minute structured interview and was developed in order to standardise and obtain information relevant to diagnostic criteria. The structured clinical interview used is the DSM-IV-R, PANSS edition (SCID-PANSS)

(Kay et al., 2006). Both patients/participants were interviewed for 30 days and one day prior to the start of the probiotic treatment and 30, 60 and 120 days after the commencement of the probiotic treatment (Nagamine et al., 2012). Faecal flora was checked from both participants using the terminal-restriction fragment length polymorphism method one day prior to the start of the probiotic treatment and 30 and 120 days after commencement of the probiotic treatment (Nagamine et al., 2012).

The study found very little change in either schizophrenia symptoms or the content of the faecal flora in both patients/participants prior to commencement of the probiotic treatment. Parallel changes were found in both the severity of schizophrenia symptoms and the faecal flora 30 days after commencement of treatment, which continued through to 120 days (Nagamine et al., 2012). There was a reduction in total PANSS scores for the patient/participant receiving probiotic treatment compared to the patient that did not receive the probiotic treatment. The main reduction was found in the severity of negative symptoms. The PANSS scores for the patient/participant that did not receive the probiotic treatment did not change during the 150 days of the study (Nagamine et al., 2012). A similar pattern of change was observed in the faecal flora of the two patients/participants. Limited change was found in the faecal flora of the patient/participant not receiving the probiotic treatment. The common pattern found in the flora for this patient was Bacteroides (30%) and an absence of Bifidobacterium. In the patient/participant that received the probiotic treatment changes in the faecal flora was found 30 days after commencement of treatment. There was a reduction in the presence of the bacterium Enterococcus from a peak of 60% of the total flora. At the same time Clostridium, Ruminococcus, Eubacterium, Catenibacterium and Bacteriodes bacterium appeared and this change continued through to the 120 day of treatment (Nagamine et al., 2012).

The authors of the study suggest that the observed parallel changes in PANSS scores and faecal flora are associated. They offer the explanation that the change in intestinal flora altered the cytokine balance, which in turn had a positive impact on the central nervous system (Nagamine et al., 2012, page 68). It is also suggested that the changes in PANSS scores and faecal flora after treatment with probiotics imply a clinical significance for immunological processes in the aetiology of schizophrenia (Nagamine et al., 2012). Whilst the findings of this study are interesting and form the basis for future studies, much more evidence from robust and well organised experimental studies are required before these claims can be substantiated.

There is a paucity of further evidence supporting the efficacy of probiotics on either the positive and negative symptoms of schizophrenia and this is due to there being so few reported studies investigating the efficacy of probiotics with this client group. There is more substantial historical and emerging evidence implicating inflammatory responses and immunological processes in the development of psychiatric conditions such as anxiety and schizophrenia symptoms (Dohan et al., 1969; Laan et al., 2010). Although this evidence does not provide support for the efficacy and suitability of probiotics for people with schizophrenia, it does identify potential causal pathways which may be sensitive to the beneficial effects of probiotics.

Microbial Endocrinology, Probiotics and Neuroactive Compounds

The term microbial endocrinology has been used to describe the study of the action of the biochemicals that influence the functioning of the immune system, gastro intestinal tract and the central and autonomic nervous systems simultaneously (Lyte, 2011). The hypothesis that emanates from microbial endocrinology about probiotics and schizophrenia symptoms is based on their ability to produce neuroactive substances, which indicates a shared therapeutic mechanism on immune, gastric and neural systems. Two neurochemicals produced by probiotics have been implicated in the development of schizophrenia symptoms (Dopamine-Bacillus Serratia and GABA-Lactobacillus Bifidobacterium) indicating a shared neurophysiological intersystem signalling by neurotransmitters implicated in the development of psychotic symptoms (Lyte, 2011). The anxiety reducing effect of Bifidobacterium Lactobacillus and Bifidiobacterium Longum (NCC3001) in both humans and rats further supports the potential benefits of specific probiotics in treating anxiety related psychotic symptoms (Bercik et al., 2011; Messaoudi et al., 2011).

The Gut–Brain Axis: Potential Aetiological Pathways for the Development of Schizophrenia Symptoms

The findings from recent animal and clinical studies have suggested that there is a neuronal and hormonal bi-directional communication between gastro intestinal disturbances, inflammatory conditions, central nervous system biochemistry, autonomic responses and behaviour (Neufeld et al., 2011; Cryan and O'Mahony, 2011).

Studies investigating stress responses in germ free mice compared to specific pathogen free mice found significant differences in behaviour characteristic of reduced anxiety in favour of the germ-free mice (Neufeld et al., 2011). This same study found significantly higher comparative levels of corticosterone levels in the germ-free mice ($t = 2.48$, $df = 22$, $p = 0.021$) as well as a significant comparative differences in the up-regulation of Brain Derived Neutrophic Factor messenger RNA in the denate gyrus of the hippocampus ($t = 2.97$, $df = 20$, $p = 0.0076$). These findings provide evidence in support of the influence of conventional intestinal flora on the physiology of the stress response (Neufeld et al., 2011). Other animal studies have found that chronic colitis was associated with increased anxiety like behaviour in male mice. The administration of the probiotic Bifidobacterium longum (NCC3001) to these mice was effective at normalising behaviour but not at reducing inflammation measured by myeloperoxidase activity (Bercik et al., 2011). Bifidobacterium longum metabolites did not increase the production of Brain Derived Neutrophic Factor in neural (SH-SY5Y) cells. The anxiolytic effect of Bifidobacterium longum was dependent on the integrity of the vagus nerve, suggesting that the vagus nerve has a key role in mediating anxiety and its related behaviour. This finding may indicate lack of direct effect of this probiotic on the central nervous system but that it may exert and influence via the vagus nerve pathway (Bercik et al., 2011). GABA is the principal inhibitory neurotransmitter, which has been linked to the development of higher levels of anxiety and depression. Change in the functioning of the GABAergic system was induced by continuous administration of the probiotic Lactobacillus rhamnosus (JB-1) to mice (Bravo et al., 2011). Reduced anxiety type behaviours in treated mice were observed in an elevated plus maze. Changes in the GABAergic system were found in the mice that received the Lactobacillus rhamnosus (JB-1) and included regional increases in $GABA_{B1b}$ mRNA in the cingulate and prelimbic cortical regions of the brain (Bravo et al., 2011). Concurrent reductions in the expression of GABA receptor were found in the amygdala, hippocampus and locus coerulues. A significant interaction was found between acute stress, treatment with Lactobacillus rhamnosus (JB-1) and corticosterone levels ($F_{(1, 28)} = 11.409$, p = 0.0022). The level of stress induced corticosterone was significantly lower in the mice that were treated with Lactobacillus rhamnosus (JB-1) (p < 0.001) (Bravo et al., 2011). Administration of Lactobacillus rhamnosus (JB-1) was found to increase $GABA_{A\alpha2}$ mRNA receptor expression in the hippocampus and was found to reduce $GABA_{A\alpha2}$ mRNA expression receptor in the prefrontal cortex and amygdala. These same changes were not found in vagotomised mice, indicating that the vagus nerve may mediate anxiety and depression and the beneficial effects of Lactobacillus rhamnosus (JB-1).

The functioning of the immune system and particularly the role of lymphocytes influencing central nervous system functioning has also been investigated. T cell deficiency in mature mice has been linked to the development of cognitive deficits and behavioural abnormalities (Kipnis et al., 2004). Stimulation of the development of T cells overcame the amphetamine induced behavioural and cognitive changes in the mature mice indicating a central role for the adaptive immune system in cognitive functioning (Kipnis et al., 2004).

O'Mahony et al. (2011) describe the gut–brain axis as a complex reflex network that is made up of receptors, neurotransmitters, afferent and efferent fibres that project into different parts of the autonomic nervous system such as integrative central areas and smooth muscle and glands. The bi-directional nature of the communication suggests that the brain can influence gastro intestinal functioning and vice versa in terms of the gastro intestinal system influencing reflex responses and regulation (O'Mahony et al., 2011). This model of communication within the axis implies that psychological processes, particularly stress responses, can influence gastro-intestinal functioning and gastro-intestinal functioning can influence cognitions, emotional response and behaviour. The Hypothalamic-pituitary axis (HPA) is activated by chronic stress and is made up of three main structures; (1) the hypothalamus, (2) the pituitary gland, and (3) the adrenal glands. The HPA regulates the immune system and is the mechanism that regulates the bio-psychological stress response in humans. Corticotrophin-releasing factor receptors produced as part of the HPA function are found in both the central nervous system and the gastro-intestinal tract. Secretion of corticotrophin-releasing factor (CRF) within the gastro-intestinal tract has been found to influence a number of functions of gut–brain axis such as transit, visceral sensation and permeability of the intestinal wall (O'Mahony et al., 2011). Providing evidence of the central role played by the HPA and its products within the gut–

brain axis (McKernan et al., 2010; Neufeld et al., 2011). A number of mechanisms and study findings have been identified as evidence supporting this gut–brain axis (O'Mahony et al., 2011).

1. The high co-morbidity found in clinical studies between stress related conditions and gastrointestinal disorders (Bercik et al., 2011; Cryan and O'Mahony, 2011).

2. Links between chronic stress and anxiety, immune response and the development of inflammatory conditions such as irritable bowel syndrome (McKernan et al., 2010; Neufeld et al., 2011).

3. Implication of the action of chronic stress on the regulation of stress response hormones initiated by the hypothalamic-pituitary-adrenal axis and its association with the development of irritable bowel syndrome (McKernan et al., 2010).

4. Associations between gastro-intestinal infections and changes in behaviour and central nervous system biochemistry such as changes in tryptophan metabolism causing and increasing levels of anxiety inducing kynurenin (Bercik et al., 2011). Alterations in the level of kynurenine 3-monooxygenase enzymes within the kynurenine pathway leading to increased concentrations of cortical kynurenic acid in the cerebrospinal fluid have been associated with the development of neuro-cognitive deficits found in people with schizophrenia (Wonodi et al., 2011).

Only minimal evidence has been developed regarding the effects of probiotics on the alleviation of schizophrenia symptoms (Nagamine et al., 2012). However, pathways linking immunological processes and the development of schizophrenia symptoms and the functioning of the HPA within the stress vulnerability model of schizophrenia symptom development, provide the framework and targets for the setting of future study hypotheses regarding the testing of efficacy of probiotics (Cryan and O'Mahony, 2011).

Schizophrenia Symptoms and Autoimmune Processes as Potential Aetiological Pathways

The role of inflammatory responses in the development of schizophrenia symptoms has been explored previously (Dohan, 1983; Laan et al., 2010). Epidemiological studies have found links between immunological responses and increased risk of developing schizophrenia (Dohan, 1946; Eaton et al., 2006). Nine autoimmune diseases (thyrotoxicosis, intestinal malabsorption, acquired haemolytic anaemia, chronic active hepatitis, interstitial cystitis, alopecia areata, myositis, polymyalgia rheumatica and Sjorgren's syndrome) had significantly higher prevalence rates amongst a birth cohort population of Danish people with a diagnosis of schizophrenia (n = 7704) compared to those without (Eaton et al., 2006). This study used participants where the autoimmune disorder had occurred before the schizophrenia symptoms had developed. Crude incidence rate ratios were reported in the study and are shown in Table 2. Having a history of autoimmune disease accounted for a 45% increased risk of developing schizophrenia.

Table 2 Crude incidence rate ratios for the nine autoimmune diseases that had higher lifetime prevalence among those diagnosed with schizophrenia compared to those without the diagnosis (Table adapted from Eaton et al., 2006).

Autoimmune disorder	Crude incidence rate	
	Ratio	95% CI
Thyrotoxicosis	2.3	1.1–4.8
Intestinal malabsorption/Celiac's disease	3.8	1.3–11.0
Acquired hemolytic anemia	12.5	3.1–50.0
Chronic active hepatitis	8.3	2.7–25.8
Interstitial cystitis	2.1	1.6–2.9
Alopecia areata	2.4	1.0–5.6
Myositis	1.9	1.4–2.7
Polymyalgia rheumatica	4.2	1.6–10.8
Sjorgren's syndrome	12.4	1.1–137.8

Eaton et al. (2006) suggest caution with some of the findings of their study. Large incidence ratio's for both acquired haemolytic anaemia and Sjorgen's syndrome were based on very small incidence rates (3 and 1). Diagnosis of the autoimmune disorders was based on diagnosis in speciality services and the authors suggest this may lead to under ascertainment as many people will not attend speciality services. The authors also point out that the onset of many autoimmune disorders is later than that for schizophrenia and may skew the findings in terms of autoimmune disorders increasing the risk of developing schizophrenia.

Explanations of the relationships between autoimmune disorders and the development of schizophrenia symptoms have focused on shared genetic vulnerability to both autoimmune disorders and schizophrenia. This shared genetic vulnerability could occur in terms of common variants causing multiple diseases including autoimmune disorders and schizophrenia or through a limited number of genes specific to the development of autoimmune disorders also being associated with the development of schizophrenia (Eaton et al., 2006). Genetic linkage and association studies have found genes common to both autoimmune disorders and schizophrenia and gene variants common to both disorders (Ye et al., 2005; Bradford et al., 2008).

Exposure to infection *in utero* has been found to increase the risk of developing schizophrenia, more recently sophisticated studies have identified specific candidate infections that predispose the infant to developing schizophrenia symptoms later in life (Brown and Derkitis, 2010). Prenatal influenza in the first trimester has been one of those candidate infections that has been associated with a seven-fold increase in risk for developing schizophrenia symptoms in a population based birth cohort. *In utero* exposure to influenza in early to mid-pregnancy was associated with a three-fold increase in risk, whereas there was no increased risk where there was exposure in the second and third trimester (Brown et al., 2004). The cellular and molecular mechanisms by which exposure increases the risk is not yet known (Brown and Derkitis, 2010).

In a well-controlled, double blind study a sample of people diagnosed with DSM-IV schizophrenia spectrum disorders (n = 70) were randomly allocated to receive either adjuvant aspirin therapy or placebo. Adjuvant aspirin therapy (1000 mg/day) was found to have beneficial effects on the presentation of both negative and positive symptoms of schizophrenia (medium effect size 0.5). The mean score difference for the total PANSS scores between the aspirin group and the placebo group after three months of treatment was significant (3.81, p = 0.018) (Laan et al., 2010). Adjuvant aspirin therapy was also associated with an increase in T_H1/T_H2 cell cytokine production. Further borderline significant associations (p = 0.05) were found between those with the lowest anti-inflammatory cytokine production and higher anti-psychotic effect as measured by the PANSS. Conversely, those with the highest anti-inflammatory cytokine production had the lowest anti-psychotic effect as measured by the PANSS (Laan et al., 2010). These findings confirm the association between inflammatory processes and the development of schizophrenia symptoms and also indicate a role for anti-inflammatory cytokines as opposed to pro-inflammatory cytokines in the amelioration of psychotic symptoms.

Vincent et al. (2011) describes a category of immunotherapy-responsive central nervous system disorders called autoimmune encephalopathies. These disorders affect one of the key neurotransmitters that have been linked to the development of schizophrenia like symptoms (Coyle et al., 2003; Coyle, 2006). N-methyl-D-aspartate receptor antibody encephalitis is a disorder where the action of autoantibodies are stimulated and used against healthy tissue. The development of this disorder has been associated with the development of a tumour and in other cases of infection (Marsland and Bray, 2012). Early presenting symptoms include headache, fever, nausea, diarrhoea and upper respiratory tract symptoms. Psychiatric symptoms include personality and behaviour changes, short term memory loss and acute psychosis including delusions and hallucinations (Marsland and Bray, 2012). Somewhere in the region of a quarter of the people that contract N-methyl-D-aspartate receptor antibody encephalitis will have longer term morbidities or unfortunately die from the disorder (Vincent et al., 2011).

HPA Functioning and the Stress Vulnerability Model Further Potential Pathways for Understanding the Impact of Probiotics on Schizophrenia Symptoms

The functioning of the hypothalamic-pituitary axis (HPA) is associated with the development of schizophrenia symptoms in a sample (n = 94) of people at high risk of developing symptoms (Garner et al., 2005; Pariante et al., 2005). Participants were observed over a one year period and pituitary volume was measured using a 1.5 mm, coronal 1.5-T high resolution magnetic resonance imager. The participants that developed schizophrenia symptoms (n = 31) were found to have a significant larger baseline pituitary volume (+12%, p < 0.001) in comparison to those participants that did not develop schizophrenia symptoms (n = 63) (Garner et al., 2005). The risk for developing schizophrenia symptoms was 20% increased risk for every 10% rise in baseline pituitary volume (Garner et al., 2005). Similar patterns of increased pituitary volume (+22%, p < 0.001) were found in a sample of people experiencing their first psychotic episode (n = 78) compared to an age and gender matched group of control participants (n = 78) (Pariante et al., 2005).

The effects of increased pituitary volume on the development of schizophrenia symptoms can be understood through the mechanisms of the stress vulnerability model (SVM) (Nuchterlein and Dawson, 1984a; Fleming and Martin, 2012). The SVM defines a temporal process that integrates a range of bio-psycho-social factors in a process that explains the development of schizophrenia symptoms (Nicholson and Neufeld, 1992). Within this temporal process maintaining equilibrium is the main outcome for the individual. The model is made up of three interacting parts; (1) vulnerability factors are those bio-psycho-social factors that individually or as a combination of factors that contribute to the likelihood of developing schizophrenia. In born vulnerability is characteristic of biological vulnerabilities such as a genetic predisposition or chemical dysregulation. Acquired vulnerability was identified as vulnerability factors that developed post birth such as trauma, interpersonal difficulties and specific diseases (Zubin and Spring, 1977). Nuchterlein and Dawson (1984a) further identified four personal vulnerability factors; dopaminergic dysregulation, information processing and attentional deficits, autonomic hyperreactivity and schizotypal personality traits. Vulnerability is individualised and each person is imbued with different levels of vulnerability. The magnitude of vulnerability determines the level of proneness to developing schizophrenia; the higher the level of vulnerability the increased risk of that person developing schizophrenia. The level of vulnerability defines the person's stress threshold or capacity to tolerate and absorb stress. (2) Stress works as a precipitating factor within the SVM. Where the person experiences a high level of stress or the cumulative effects of stress which breaches the persons predetermined stress threshold. This means that the stress cannot be absorbed and the person's vulnerability will express itself in the development of schizophrenia symptoms in those sufficiently vulnerable. If the stress remains below the predetermined stress threshold the person will not develop schizophrenia symptoms. (3) Mediating factors are personal and environmental coping and resilience factors that influence the development of schizophrenia symptoms in those imbued with sufficient vulnerability (Nuchterlein and Dawson, 1984a). The development of good pre-morbid functioning, confidence, self-esteem, social networks and coping ability can protect against the development of schizophrenia by facilitating with the absorption of stress or by increasing the person's stress threshold (Fleming and Martin, 2012).

Central to the temporal process (see Figure 1) is the concept of the prodromal period. Within this period information processing overloads occur as a consequence of the interaction between personal vulnerability factors and personal and environmental stressors. High levels of autonomic physiological arousal is a crucial part of the process, which further exacerbates the persons information processing difficulties, reduces their ability to cope effectively with stress and contributes to the activation of schizophrenia symptoms (Nuchterlein and Dawson, 1984b; Fleming and Martin, 2012). Increased pituitary volume and changes within the HPA could explain the mechanisms of physiological hyperarousal and how this translates into the development of schizophrenia symptoms in the prodromal period. Autonomic hyperreactivity is a personal vulnerability factor and also provides a potential explanation for the role of increased pituitary volume and changes in HPA functioning in the development of schizophrenia symptoms.

Activation of the HPA appears to be consistent with the development of schizophrenia symptoms (Pariante et al., 2005) and the hormones and peptides secreted by the structures within the HPA are also associated with the functioning of the gastro intestinal system and the gut brain axis (O'Mahony et al., 2011). The gut brain axis involves bi-directional communication between structures and their products within the gastro intestinal system, the immune system, the central nervous system and autonomic nervous system. Probiotics influence this interactive bio-immune-neurophysiological environment. Findings that support the links between the HPA and gut brain axis provide evidence of the potential suitability of pathways linked to the development of schizophrenia symptoms that may be susceptible to the effects of probiotics (Lyte, 2011).

Conclusions

Implications for clinical practice

The evidence base supporting the beneficial effects of probiotics on reducing schizophrenia is limited to one case study (Nagamine et al., 2012). Case study evidence provides data that can influence the design of future studies but does not provide equivocal evidence to guide clinical practice. Evidence from wider populations indicate that specific strains of probiotics can confer beneficial anxiolytic and immunological effects on the host (Toedter-Williams, 2010). Both of these effects would be particularly salient for people that experience high levels of physiological arousal and/or receive anti-psychotic pharmaceutical treatment. The temporal process described within the structure of the stress vulnerability suggest that schizophrenia symptoms emerge through a predisposition to increased autonomic hyperreactivity and physiological arousal, which combine to activate personal vulnerabilities that emerge as schizophrenia symptoms (Nuchterlein and Dawson, 1984a). This process is likely exacerbated by increased activity of the HPA (Pariante et al., 2005). The gut–brain axis supports the transfer of beneficial effects from the gastro intestinal tract through to anxiolytic effects via probiotics (McKernan et al., 2010; Cryan and O'Mahony, 2011; Neufeld et al., 2011). The anxiolytic effects of probiotics may well mediate the effects of the relationship between stress and vulnerabilities and consequently reduce the risk of this relationship activating vulnerabilities and schizophrenia symptoms from developing. The side effects of pharmaceutical anti-psychotic treatment can influence the immunological system of the host (Chen et al., 2011). The immunological effects of probiotics may be beneficial in supporting the immune system of those people requiring long term anti-psychotic medication.

Implications for future research

Presently these potential benefits of probiotics are only theoretical and require empirical support. Double blind randomised controlled trails provide the most effective and robust study design to determine cause and effect (Portney and Watkins, 2009) between specific strains of probiotic such as Bifidobacterium Lactobacillus,

Bifidiobacterium Longum (NCC3001) and Lactobacillus rhamnosus (JB-1) and an anxiolytic effect and reduction in schizophrenia symptoms in those people with the diagnosis (Bercik et al., 2011; Bravo et al., 2011). The stress vulnerability model can provide the template and framework by which well-designed trials can measure the potential anti-psychotic and anxiolytic effects of specific strains of probiotics. HPA and GABAergic functioning fits within the template of the stress vulnerability model as potential physiological vulnerability factors and/or part of the process of increasing hyperarousal (Nuchterlein and Dawson, 1984a) and would be suitable targets for designing outcomes measures for studies investigating the potential anxiolytic effects of probiotics.

References

American Psychiatric Association (1994) Diagnostic Criteria from the DSM-IV. Washington, DC: American Psychiatric Association.

Andreasen NC (1982) Negative symptoms in schizophrenia. Definition and reliability. Archives of Gerontology and Geriatrics 39(7): 784–788.

Bentall RP (2009) Doctoring the Mind: Why Psychiatric Treatments Fail. Penguin Psychology, London.

Bercik P, Park AJ, Sinclair D, Khoshdel A, Lu J, Huang X, Deng Y, Blennerhaussett PA, Fahnestock M, Moine D, Berger B, Huizinga JD, Kunze W, Mclean PG, Bergonzelli GE, Collins SM and Verdu EF (2011) The anxiolytic effect of Bifidobacterium longum NCC3001 involves vagal pathways for gut–brain communication. Neurogastroenterology and Motility 23: 1132–1154.

Bleuler E (1911) Dementia Praecox or the Group of Schizophrenias (translated by J. Zinkin), New York, International Universities Press.

Bradford M, Law MH, Stewart AD, Shaw DJ, Megson IL and We J (2008) The TGM2 gene is associated with schizophrenia in a British population. American Journal of Medical Genetics, part B, Neuropyschiatric Genetics 150B: 335–340.

Bravo JA, Forsythe P, Chew MV, Escaravage E, Savignac HM, Dinan TG, Bienstock J and Cryan JF (2011) Ingestion of Lactobacillus strain regulates emotional behaviour and central GABA receptor expression in a mouse via the vagus nerve. www.pnas.org/cgi/doi/10.1073/pnas.1102999108.

Brown AS, Begg MD, Gravenstein S, Schaefer CA, Wyatt RJ, Bresnahan M, Babulas VP and Susser ES (2004) Serologic evidence of prenatal influenza in the etiology of schizophrenia. Archives of Gerontology and Geriatrics 61(8): 774–780.

Brown AS and Derkitis EJ (2010) Prenatal infection and schizophrenia: a review of epidemiological and translational studies. American Journal of Psychiatry 167(3): 261–280.

Chen ML, Tsai TC, Lin YY, Tsai YM, Wang LK, Lee MC and Tsai FM (2011) Antipsychotic drugs suppress the AKT/NF-κB pathway and regulate the differentiation of T-cell subsets. Immunology Letters 140(1-2): 81–91.

Clare A (1976) Psychiatry in Dissent. Controversial Issues in Thought and Practice (2nd edition). Routledge, London, Tavistock.

Coyle JT, Tsai G and Goff D (2003) Converging evidence of NMDA receptor hypofunction in the pathophysiology of schizophrenia. Annals of the New York Academy of Sciences 1003: 318–327.

Coyle JT (2006) Glutamate and schizophrenia: beyond the dopamine hypothesis. Cellular and Molecular Neurobiology 26(4-6): 365–384.

Crow TJ (1980) Molecular pathology of schizophrenia: more than one disease process? British Medical Journal 280(6207): 66–68.

Crow TJ (1985) The Two-syndrome concept: Origins and current status. Schizophrenia Bulletin 11(2): 471–485.

Cryan JF and O'Mahony SM (2011) The microbiome-gut–brain axis: from bowel to behaviour. Neurogastroenterology and Motility 23: 187–192.

Dohan FC (1946) Wartime changes in hospital admissions for schizophrenia. A comparison of admission for schizophrenia and other psychoses in six countries during World War II. Acta Psychiatrica Scandinavica 42: 1–23.

Dohan FC, Grasberger J, Lowell FM, Johnston HT and Arbegast AW (1969) Relapsed Schizophrenics: More rapid improvement on a milk- and cereal-free diet. British Journal of Psychiatry 115: 595–596.

Dohan FC (1983) More on Celiac Disease as a model for schizophrenia. Biological Psychiatry 18: 561–564.

Eaton WW, Byrne M, Ewald H, Mors O, Chen CY, Agerbo E and Mortensen PB (2006) Association of schizophrenia and autoimmune diseases: linkage of danish national registers. American Journal of Psychiatry 163(3): 521–528.

Fleming M and Martin CR (2012) From classical psychodynamics to evidence synthesis; the motif of repression and a contemporary understanding of a key mediatory mechanism in psychosis. Current Psychiatry Reports 14(3): 252–258.

Garner B, Pariante CM, Wood SJ, Velakoulis D, Phillips L, Soulsby B, Brewer WJ, Smith DJ, Dazzan P, Berger GE, Yung AR, van den Buuse M, Murray R, McGorry PD and Pantelis C (2005) Pituitary volume predicts future transition to psychosis in individuals at ultra-high risk of developing psychosis. Biological Psychiatry 58: 417–423.

Goldstein J and Kreisma D (1988) Gender, family environment and schizophrenia. Psychological Medicine 18: 861–872.

Goldstein J and Lewine R (2000) Overview of sex differences in schizophrenia. pp. 111–143. In: Castle D, McGrath J and Kulkharni J (Eds.). Women and Schizophrenia. Cambridge University Press.

Harding CM, Brooks GW, Ashikaga T, Strauss JS and Breier A (1987) The Vermont longitudinal study of persons with severe mental illness, II: Long-term outcome of subjects who retrospectively met DSM-III criteria for schizophrenia. American Journal of Psychiatry 144(6): 727–735.

Kay S, Opler L and Lindenmayer J (1989) The Positive and Negative Syndrome Scale (PANSS): Rationale and standardisation. British Journal of Psychiatry 155: 59–65.

Kay S, Opler LA and Fizbein A (2006) Positive and Negative Syndrome Scale: Technical Manual. Multi-Health Systems Inc. Tonawanda, New Jersey.

Kendell R and Jablensky A (2003) Distinguishing between the validity and utility of psychiatric diagnoses. American Journal of Psychiatry 160(1): 4–12.

Kipnis J, Cohen H, Cardon ZY and Schwartz M (2004) T cell deficiency leads to cognitive dysfunction: Implications of therapeutic vaccination for schizophrenia and other psychiatric conditions. www.pnas.org/cgi/doi/10.1073/pnas.0402268101.

Kraepelin E (1913) Dementia Praecox. In: Kraepelin E (Ed.). Psychiatrica, 8th edition (translated by R. Barclay). Melbourne.

Krieger FL, Laan W, Grobbee DE, Selten J-P, Heijnen CJ, Kahn RS and Burger H (2010) Adjuvant aspirin therapy reduces symptoms of schizophrenia spectrum disorders: Results from a randomised, double-blind, placebo-controlled trial. Journal of Clinical Psychiatry 71(5): 520–527.

Laan W, Grobee DE, Selten JP, Heijnen CJ, Kahn RS and Burger H (2010) Adjuvant aspirin therapy reduces symptoms of schizophrenia spectrum disorders: results from a randomised, double-blind, placebo-controlled trial. Journal of Clinical Psychiatry 71(5): 520–527. doi 10.4088/JCP.09m05117yel.

Lyte M (2011) Probiotics function mechanistically as delivery vehicles for neuroactive compounds: Microbial endocrinology in the design and use of probiotics. www.bioessays-journal.com. Wiley Periodicals, Inc.

Martin CR and Fleming M (2009) Issues in Quality of life assessment in schizophrenia. In: Preedy VR and Watson RR (Eds.). Handbook of Disease Burdens and Quality of Life Measures. Springer, Germany.

Marsland L and Bray J (2012) Anti-NMDA receptor antibody encephalitis: a new challenge in the diagnosis of psychosis. British Journal of Neuroscience Nursing 8(5): 276–281.

McKernan DP, Fitzgerald P, Dinan TG and Cryan JF (2010) The probiotic Bifidobacterium infantis 35624 displays visceral antinociceptive effects in the rat. Neurogastroenterology & Motility 22: 1029–1035.

Messaoudi M, Lalonde R, Violle N, Javelot H and Rougeot C (2011) Assessment of psychotropic like properties of a probiotic formulation (Lactobacillus helveticus R0052 and bifidiobacteruim longum R0175 in rats and human subjects. British Journal of Nutrition 105: 755–774.

Nagamine T, Sato N and Seo G (2012) Probiotics reduce negative symptoms of schizophrenia: A case report. Internal Medicine Journal 19(1): 62–68.

Neufeld KM, Kang N, Bienstock J and Foster JA (2011) Reduced anxiety-like behaviour and central neurochemical change in germ-free mice. Neurogastroenterology & Motility 23: 255–264.

Nicholson I and Neufeld W (1992) A dynamic vulnerability perspective on stress and psychosis. American Journal of Orthopsychiatry 62(1): 117–129.

Nuchterlein KH and Dawson ME (1984a) A heuristic vulnerability/stress model of schizophrenic episodes. Schizophrenia Bulletin 10: 300–312.

Nuchterlein KH and Dawson ME (1984b) Information processing and attentional functioning in the developmental course of schizophrenia. Schizophrenia Bulletin 10: 160–203.

O'Mahony S, Hyland NP, Dinan TG and Cryan JF (2011) Maternal separation as a model of brain–gut axis dysfunction. Psychopharmacology 214: 71–88.

Pariante CM, Dazzan P, Danese A, Morgan KD, Brudaglio F, Morgan C, Fearon P, Orr K, Hutchinson G, Pantelis C, Velakoulis D, Jones PB, Leff J and Murray RM (2005) Increased pituitary volume in antipsychotic-free and antipsychotic-treated patients of the Aesop first-onset psychosis study. Neuropsychopharmacology 30(10): 1923–1931.

Portney LG and Watkins MP (2009) Foundations of Clinical Research: Applications to Practice (3rd edition). Upper Saddle River, NJ, Prentice-Hall.

Rajji TK, Ismail Z and Mulsant BH (2009) Age at onset and cognition in schizophrenia: meta-analysis. British Journal of Psychiatry 195: 286–293.

Reid G, Jass J Sebulsky and McCormick MT (2003) Potential uses of probiotics in clinical practice. Clinical Microbiology Reviews 16(4): 658–672.

Santosa S, Farnworth E and Jones P (2006) Probiotics and their potential health claims. Nutrition Reviews 64: 265–274.

Tandon R, Keshavan MS and Nasrallah HA (2008) Schizophrenia, "Just the facts". What we know in 2008. Part 1: Overview. Schizophrenia Research 100: 4–19.

Toedter-Williams N (2010) Probiotics. American Journal of Health-System Pharmacy 67: 449–458.

Vincent A, Bie CG, Irani SR and Waters P (2011) Autoantibodies associated with diseases of the CNS: new developments and future challenges. Lancet 10(8): 759–772.

Weichselbaum E (2010) Reviewing the data on the effects of probiotics. Practice Nursing 21(1): 14–16.

Wonodi I, Stine C, Sathyasaikumar KV, Roberts RC, Mitchell BD, Hong LE, Kajit Y, Thaker GK and Schwartz R (2011) Downregulated kynurenine 3-monooxygenase gene expression and enzyme activity in schizophrenia and genetic association with schizophrenia endophenotypes. Archives of Gerontology and Geriatrics 68(7): 665–674.

World Health Organisation (1992) The International Classification of Diseases-10 Mental and behavioural disorders. Geneva: Switzerland: World Health Organisation.

World Health Organisation (2002) Guidelines for the evaluation of probiotics in food. Report of a joint FAO/WHO working group. London, Ontario, Canada: FAO/WHO.

Ye L, Wei J, Sun Z, Xie L, Liu S, Ju G, Shi J, Yu Y, Zhang X and Xu Q (2005) Further study of a genetic association between the CLDN5 locus and schizophrenia. Schizophrenia Research 75(1): 139–141.

Zubin J and Spring B (1977) Vulnerability: a new view of schizophrenia. Journal of Abnormal Psychology 86: 260–266.

Chapter 12

Probiotics and Alzheimer's Disease

Derek Larkin[1,]* and *Colin R Martin*[2]

INTRODUCTION

There are thought to be 44 million people in the world suffering from dementia, including Alzheimer's disease (Latypova and Martin, 2014). By 2030 it is estimated that 66 million people will be living with dementia and by 2050 that number will have grown to 115 million people (Prince et al., 2013). Alzheimer's disease accounts for 60 to 80% of all dementia. Dementia has been described as one of the most challenging medical problems facing aging communities across the globe, and despite enormous efforts to combat the condition, a medical cure remains frustratingly elusive (Alzheimer's Association, 2017; Jiang et al., 2017).

The yearly monetary cost of dementia for individuals living with the condition and who depend on care provision in the United States, has been estimated to be around $70,000. This amounts to a total national health care bill of $157 billion to $215 billion (Hurd et al., 2013). As dementia affects an ever-increasing aging population, it represents a substantial social and economic burden across all societies, similar in size and scope to that of heart disease and cancer (Hurd et al., 2013).

Dementia is a chronic disease of aging characterized by the progression of cognitive decline that interferes with every aspect of the person's independent function (American Psychiatric Association, 2013). Dementia should not be thought of as a single entity but instead as a syndrome, in which there are many symptoms, each with several causes (see Figure 1). Characteristically dementia includes difficulties with memory, language, problem solving and other cognitive skills that affect the

[1] Edge Hill University, St Helens Road, Ormsirk, Lancashire, L39 4QP.
[2] Faculty of Society and Health, Buckinghamshire New University, Uxbridge Campus, 106 Oxford Road, Uxbridge, Middlesex, UB8 1NA, UK.
* Corresponding author

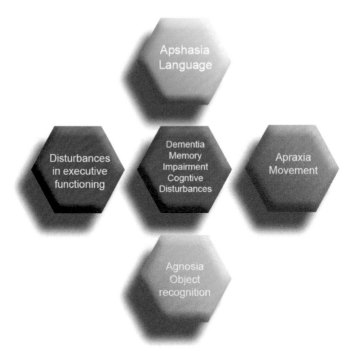

Figure 1 Loss of cognitive skills often observed in dementia.

person's ability to perform everyday activities (Alzheimer's Association, 2017). The cognitive decline can be mapped through neuronal degeneration; first to be affected are the cognitive areas of the brain, for example the hippocampus making the coding and retrieval of memories difficult. Eventually the dementia spreads to other regions of the brain, damaging neurons and compromising function. From the hippocampus, the damage spreads to the language centres of the brain making retrieval and production of words difficult. The disorder affects the areas of the brain involved in logical thought, making the ability to solve problems, grasp concepts and making plans difficult. The illness will invariably effect the areas of the brain involved in emotion, the patient may lose the ability to control their mood and feelings. The condition may also compromise the patient's ability to make sense of what they hear, see and smell, and may spark hallucinations. The condition goes on to erase the oldest memories the person may have, before it attacks the person's balance and co-ordination. Eventually Alzheimer's disease will compromise the person's ability to breathe. The progression from mild forgetting to the person's death has an average time course of 8–10 years.

The neuropathological hallmarks of Alzheimer's disease include extracellular amyloid ß, senile plaques and intracellular neurofibrillary tangles (Reitz et al., 2011). It is generally accepted that there is an interaction between genetics and environmental factors that takes place in Alzheimer's disease pathogenesis. However, recent studies suggest a significant correlation between changes in gut microbiota and cognitive behaviour (Hu et al., 2016). It has been shown that modulation of gut microbiota, using probiotics or antibiotics, faecal microbiota transplantation can modulate the hosts cognitive behaviour.

Dementia

When an individual first shows signs of dementia, and the clinician attempts to identify the cause, there can be brain abnormalities associated with more than one cause of dementia (Schneider et al., 2007; Schneider et al., 2009; Viswanathan et al., 2009 see Table 1). Different causes of dementia are associated with different but distinct patterns of brain abnormalities (see Table 2). Figure 1, illustrates the interconnectivity of dementia with cognitive features, such as, disturbances in executive function, language, movement, and object recognition difficulties.

Table 1 DSM-5 criteria for major and mild neurocognitive disorders.

DSM-5 criteria for major and mild neurocognitive disorders (previously called dementia, delirious amnesiac and other cognitive disorders)
A. Evidence of significant cognitive decline from a previous level of performance in one or more cognitive domains: a)   Learning and memory b)   Language c)   Executive function d)   Complex attention e)   Perceptual-motor f)   Social cognition
B. The cognitive deficits interfere with independence in everyday activities (i.e., at a minimum, assistance should be required with complex instrumental activities of daily living, such as paying bills or managing medications
C. The cognitive deficits do not occur exclusively in the context of a delirium
D. The cognitive deficits are not better explained by another mental disorder (e.g., major depressive disorder, schizophrenia)

Source DSM-5 (American Psychiatric Association, 2013)

Alzheimer's Disease

Alzheimer's disease was first described in 1906, but it took 70 years before it was recognized as a common cause of dementia, and a major cause of death (Alzheimer's Association, 2017; Katzman, 1976). Research into the causes of Alzheimer's disease have lead researchers down many avenues but the precise biological changes that cause the disease, and why it progresses much faster in some and not others has eluded the scientific community so far. The differences between typical age-related cognitive changes and signs of Alzheimer's disease can sometimes be extremely subtle (see Figure 2), and can sometimes be hard to spot. However the most common initial symptom is a gradually worsening ability to remember new information (Alzheimer's Association, 2017).

Table 2 Causes and characteristics of dementia.

Causes	Characteristics

Alzheimer's disease: DSM-5 major or mild cognitive disorder due to Alzheimer's disease (American Psychiatric Association, 2013, pp. 611–614)	Alzheimer's disease is the most common cause of dementia: and accounts for 60–80% percent of all dementia cases. About 50% of these cases have mixed pathology. Individuals will display a range of cognitive deficits, including mood disorders, depending on the progression of the condition, e.g., difficulty remembering names and events, communication impairment disorientation confusion, poor judgement, behaviour changes and, finally difficulty speaking, swallowing and walking.
	 Diagnostic criteria: Probable Alzheimer's disease is diagnosed if either of the following is present –
	 A. Evidence of causative Alzheimer's disease genetic mutations of family history or genetic testing
	 B. All 3 of the following are present
	   1. Clear evidence of declining memory and learning
	   2. Steady progressive, gradual decline in cognition, without extended plateaus
	   3. No evidence of mixed aetiology—neurodegenerative or cerebrovascular disease, or other neurological, mental, or systematic disease or condition likely to contribute to cognitive decline.

Major or mild vascular cognitive disorder (Vascular dementia) (American Psychiatric Association, 2013, pp. 621–624; O'Brien and Thomas, 2015)	Vascular dementia is one the most common causes of dementia after Alzheimer's disease—estimated to cause around 15% of all cases. There are currently no licensed treatments for vascular dementia. It has been noted that there is a certain amount of controversy over the exact nature between cerebrovascular pathology and cognitive impairments and the scarcity of identifiable traceable treatment targets.
	 Diagnostic criteria:
	 A. The criteria are met for major or mild cognitive disorder
	 B. The clinical features are consistent with vascular aetiology, as suggested by either of the following
	   1. Onset of cognitive deficit is temporarily related to one or more cerebrovascular events.
	   2. Evidence for decline is prominent in complex attention (including processing speed) and frontal-executive function
	 C. There is evidence of the presence of cerebrovascular disease from history, physical examination, and/or neuroimaging considered significant to account for the neurocognitive deficits
	 D. The symptoms are not better explained by another brain disease or systemic disorder
	 The diagnostic process is very dependent on structural neuroimaging—such as Magnetic Resonance Imaging (MRI) or Computerised Tomography (CT) scan.

Table 2 contd. ...

... Table 2 contd.

Causes	Characteristics

Major mild neurocognitive disorders with Lewy Bodies (McKeith et al., 2004)	Dementia with Lewy bodies is probably the second most prevalent cause of degenerative dementia in older people—only Alzheimer's disease is more common. Dementia with Lewy bodies, was only fully recognised two decades ago.
	A. The criteria are met for major or mild cognitive disorders
	B. The disorder has insidious onset and gradual progression
	C. The disorder meets a combination of core diagnostic features suggestive diagnostic features for either probable for all possible neurocognitive disorders with Lewy bodies
	  1. Core diagnostic features
	    a. Fluctuating cognition pronounced variations in attention and alertness
	    b. Recurrent visual hallucinations that were well formed and detailed
	    c. Spontaneous features of Parkinsonism, with onset subsequence to development of cognitive decline.
	  2. Suggestive diagnostic features
	    a. Meeting criteria for rapid eye movement sleep disorder
	    b. Severe neuroleptic sensitivity
	D. The disturbance is not best explained by cerebrovascular disease, another neurodegenerative disease, the effects of a substance or other mental, neurological, or systemic disorder

Mixed dementia	This disorder is characterised by the hallmark abnormalities of more than one type of dementia, most commonly seen Alzheimer's combined with vascular dementia, or Alzheimer's with dementia with Lewy bodies

Major or mild frontotemporal cognitive disorder (American Psychiatric Association, 2013; Rabinovici and Miller, 2010)	Probable frontotemporal cognitive disorder is diagnosed in either of the following is present.
	  1. Evidence of a causative frontotemporal neurocognitive disorder genetic mutation, from either family history or genetic testing
	  2. Evidence of disproportionate frontal and/or temporal lobe involvement in neuroimaging

Major or mild neurocognitive disorder due to Parkinson's disease (American Psychiatric Association, 2013, pp. 636–638)	A. Criteria are met with a major or mild cognitive disorder
	B. The disturbance occurs in this setting of established Parkinson's disease
	C. There is insidious onset and gradual progression of impairment
	D. The neurocognitive disorder is not attributable to another medical condition and is not better explained by another mental disorder
	The major or mild neurocognitive disorder is probably due to Parkinson's disease should be diagnosed if 1 and 2 are both met. The major or mild neurocognitive disorder is possibly due to Parkinson's disease should be diagnosed if 1 or 2 are both met.
	  1. There is no evidence of mixed aetiology for example absence of other neurodegenerative or cerebrovascular disease or another neurological, mental, or systemic disease or condition is likely contributed to cognitive decline
	  2. The Parkinson's disease clearly precedes the onset of neurocognitive disorder

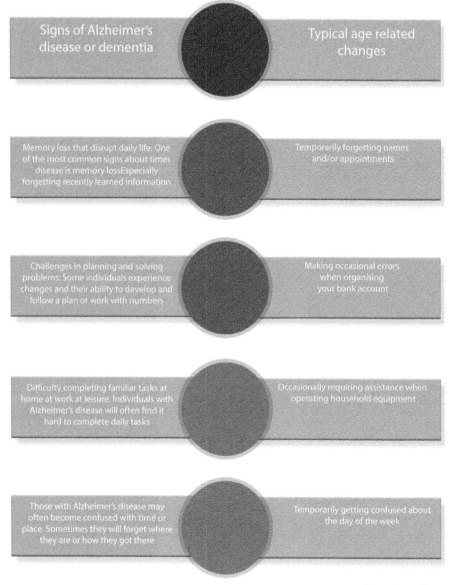

Figure 2 contd. ...

... Figure 2 contd.

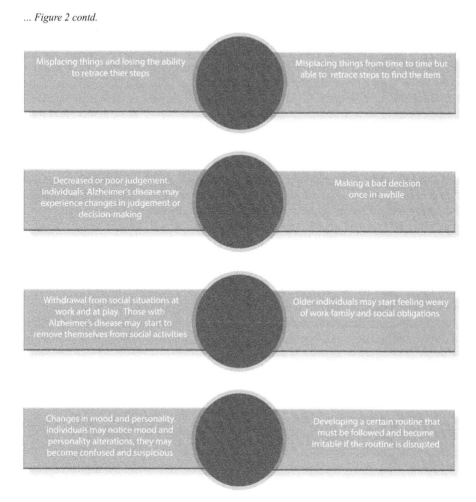

Figure 2 Signs of Alzheimer's disease or dementia versus typical age related changes.

Gut Microbiota—Life Stages

Globally life expectancy has increased at the rate of more than 3 years per decade since the 1950s (apart from the 1990s), with the exception of a few developing countries and countries emerging from economic stagnation, life expectancy has increased in most regions from 2000 onwards. Life expectancy across the globe has increased by five years between 2000 and 2015 with a 9.4 year increase in WHO African regions (World Health Organization, 2016). Life expectancy at the age of 60 has increased globally from 18.7 years in 2000 to 20.4 years in 2015. As of 2015 most individuals around the globe are expected to reach the age of 71.4 years, with individuals in most industrialised countries attaining an average life expectancy of 80 years or higher (Switzerland, Spain, Italy, Iceland, Israel, France, and Sweden). However, 22 countries have a life expectancy below the age of 60 all of them in sub Saharan Africa (World Health Organization, 2016). On average, women will live longer than men in every country of the world, and in every WHO region, female life expectancy is 73.8 years where as the male life expectancy is 69.1 years. This however, only paints a partial picture, populations can also be divided into healthy life expectancy. The WHO has also mapped years lost due to disability, and what they describe as the 'global burden of disease'. Healthy life expectancy is estimated at 63.1 years for both sexes combined. Although healthy life expectancy invariably differs between countries, on average healthy life expectancy is 11.7% shorter than life expectancy, which means for many individuals there will be a period of ill-health towards the later part of their lives.

In healthy adults, microbial communities colonise different regions of the colon that distribute nutrients and energy to the host via fermentation of non-digestible dietary components in the large intestine. Under normal circumstances this delicate balance of microbial species helps maintain a healthy metabolism and immune function. However, when this equilibrium is disrupted it can lead to negative consequences resulting in elevated inflammation and infection that have been known to contribute to metabolic disorders including inflammatory bowel disease (Frank et al., 2007), irritable bowel disease (Jeffery et al., 2012), diabetes, cardiovascular disease, colorectal cancer (Duncan and Flint, 2013; Flint, 2011; Russell et al., 2013). Evidence is starting to emerge which suggests that microbial balance may become distressed as an individual approach's old age, which may have an important role in disease pathology.

The microbial composition of the gastrointestinal tract in humans undergoes remarkable changes across the entire lifespan (O'Toole and Claesson, 2010). A neonate's gastrointestinal tract is colonised by bacteria from the mother and environment, during the birthing process and shortly after following birth. The mode of colonisation would depend to a large extent on the mode of delivery and feeding regime. Vaginal delivered infants acquired bacterial communities resembling the mother's own vaginal microbiota, which is dominated by *lactobacillus*, *Prevotella* or *Sneathia* spp., whereas infants born via Caesarian-section harbour bacterial communities similar to those found on the skin surface, dominated by *Staphylococcus*, *Corynebacterium*, and *Propionibacterium* spp. (Biasucci et al., 2010; Dominguez-Bello et al., 2010). Breast fed infants tend to harbour *Bifidobacteria* in their gastrointestinal tract whereas bottle-fed infants tend to have a much more diverse population of microbiota (Heavey et al., 2003). Once the infant is introduced to solid food the gastrointestinal environment increasingly developed towards that of adults with increased diversity (Duncan and Flint, 2013).

In a healthy adult, the colon is populated with around 10^{14} bacterial cells, outnumbering host cells tenfold, and possessing approximately 150-times as many genes as the human genome. On the whole most healthy adults have relatively stable microbial community in their colon, although there are known geographical variation in dominant phylotypes (De Filippo et al., 2010). This appears to show that there is a long-term impact on gut microbiota composition in relation to regional diets; it may also show that there are further modulations by short-term dietary changes (Duncan et al., 2007).

Studies have found that microbiota diversity declines in the elderly, with lower numbers of *Bifidobacteria* and increases in *Enterobacteriaceae* (Woodmansey, 2007) and certain *Proteobacteria*, which are suspected to play a role in the causation of bowel disease (Roberts et al., 2010). Duncan and Flint (2013) argue that the composition of the gut microbiota in the elderly, alongside metabolic activity, will to a large extent change metabolite profiles. The composition and metabolic activity of the gut microbiota appears to have a major role in contributing to health maintenance and prevention of certain diseases, as such factors that change or compromise the composition of this highly complex ecosystem are important to consider. Mortalities as a consequence of gastrointestinal infections are several times higher in the elderly compared to young adults. As such helping to maintain gut microbial balance in the elderly, may be an important objective in order to prevent disease risk (Duncan and Flint, 2013).

Probiotics and the Elderly

The word probiotics means "for (or pro) life". The World Health Organisation coined the following definition for probiotics "probiotics are live microorganisms, which, when administered in adequate amount, confer a health benefit on the host." Probiotics are food ingredients to pass through our digestive system without digestion from the host. They alter the composition or metabolism of the gut microbiota in a beneficial way, by serving as nutrients to gastrointestinal bacteria. The majority studies focus on Gram Positive *Lactobacilli* and *Bifidobacteria*, while others have concerned themselves with *Escherichia*. Among the many benefits of consuming *Bifidobacteria* include the ability to synthesise vitamins into folates (folic acid and vitamin B9). The end point of fermentation includes acetate and lactate, known to inhibit pathogens (Kleerebezem and Vaughan, 2009; Toward et al., 2012). Interestingly, studies have found that *Bifidobacteria* decreases significantly in the elderly (Claesson et al., 2012). The administration of *Bifidobacterium* species however resulted in an increased abundance of organisms in stool samples, increase in digestive transit, and reduced inflammatory status (Duncan and Flint, 2013; Ouwehand et al., 2008). On the whole, choice of probiotics used in large-scale industrial production has been based on two perceptions; the ability to confer technological advantage rather than deliver clear health benefits, the other more mundanely, is the suitability and viability during processing long-term storage. The gut is sometime seen a passive component that is victim to other age-related physiological processes, but it has been argued by Biagi et al. (2013) that alongside the other age-related physiological processes, composition of gut microbiota may determine how a human being will age. How these processes link to wellbeing of ageing individuals and longevity is still partly an open question however.

Gut Microbiome, Probiotics, and Alzheimer's Disease

It is estimated that the human brain weighs roughly equal to that of the gut (Sampson and Mazmanian, 2015). Trillions of microorganisms colonise the mammalian gastrointestinal tract from birth. These microbiota modulates development homoeostasis of the central nervous system through immune, circulatory, and neural pathways (Bauer et al., 2016; Dinan and Cryan, 2016). There is thought to be a symbiotic bidirectional communication largely involving the endocrine, immune and neural pathways (Cryan and Dinan, 2012). Up till very recently the relationship between the gut and the brain was largely ignored, however, over the past few decades increasing emphasis has been placed on the role of intestinal microbiota in regulating the gut–brain axis (Dinan and Cryan, 2016). Evidence is starting to build which indicates that microbes modulate the distance and complex centres of the central nervous system, and in turn the central nervous system exerts a top-down regulation, shaping gut physiology and microbial composition via the hypothalamic-pituitary axis (HPA).

Figure 3 illustrates the proposed mechanisms of the bi-directional gut–brain axis. (A) increased permeability which enables microbes or microbial to enter the bloodstream. (B) Gut microbes produce neurotransmitters (e.g., serotonin) and hormones (peptide PYY), in which it is suggested may impact on the hosts health. (C) Vagus nerve may directly interact via bi-directional interactions between the enteric and central nervous system. (D) There may also be gut–brain interactions as a consequence of immune-mediated inflammatory pathways. (E) Gut microbes can metabolize xenobiotics, which may impact on neurological function (Tremlett et al., 2017). There is an increasing body of research that indicates interactions between the host, the brain, and the microbiome (Bauer et al., 2016; Dinan and Cryan, 2016; Sampson and Mazmanian, 2015).

Alzheimer's disease (dementia or cognitive disorder) is amongst the most prevalent central nervous degenerative disease in the elderly. As the elderly are living much longer than previous generations, the incidences of Alzheimer's disease are set to increase exponentially (Akbari et al., 2016; Hu et al., 2016).

The pathogenesis of Alzheimer's disease is generally thought of as an interaction between genetics and environmental factors. Apolipoprotein E (ApoE) is one of the most common genetic markers for Alzheimer's disease. The gene ApoE is polymorphic with three major alleles ApoE2, ApoE3 and ApoE4 (Ghebranious et al., 2005). ApoE2 is associated with both increased and decreased risk of atherosclerosis (Breslow et al., 1982). ApoE3 is considered a neutral ApoE genotype. ApoE4 however, is implicated in atherosclerosis (Mahley, 1988) impaired cognitive function (Deary et al., 2002) reduced hippocampal volume (Farlow et al., 2004) progression in multiple sclerosis (Chapman et al., 2001) and Alzheimer's disease (Corder et al., 1993; Reitz et al., 2011). Alongside the genetic predisposition, some non-genetic factors affect the risk of Alzheimer's disease, which may include occupations where

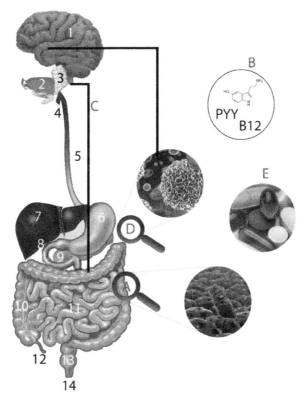

Figure 3 Adapted from https://www.britannica.com/science/human-digestive-system and Tremlett et al. (2017, p. 370). (A) Altered gut permeability, (B) Production of neuromodulator compounds, (C) Vagus nerve activation, (D) Immune pathways, (E) Microbial metabolism.

1. Human Brain, 2. Tongue, 3. Saliva Glands, 4. Pharynx, 5. Oesophagus, 6. Stomach, 7. Liver, 8. Gallbladder, 9. Pancreas, 10. Large Intestines, 11. Small Intestines, 12. Appendix, 13. Rectum, 14. Anus.

the individual encounters hazardous materials, also physical disease and lifestyle are also considered important factors. It is clear that ageing, family history and genes are important considerations in relation to the onset of Alzheimer's disease, however it has been suggested that environmental factors are more important than these other factors (Hu et al., 2016). Recent studies have suggested that human symbiotic microbes are very important factors in relation to an individual's health. The vast majority of the symbiotic microbes (95%) are located in the gut and play a major role in human nutrition, digestion, neurotrophy, inflammation, growth, immunity, and protection against pathogen infection (Hooper and Gordon, 2001; Hu et al., 2016). Composition of gut microbiota has been implicated in a number of serious conditions which include obesity (Isolauri, 2017; Ley et al., 2006), diabetes (Tilg and Moschen, 2014) hypertension (Li et al., 2017) liver cirrhosis (Qin et al., 2014; Tilg et al., 2016) autism (Finegold et al., 2010) depression (Naseribafrouei et al., 2014) Parkinson's disease (Scheperjans et al., 2015) oral cancer (Meurman, 2010) the list is seemingly endless. However, research on Alzheimer's disease and gut microbiota is in its infancy. But because of the existing research based on epidemiological investigations of Alzheimer's disease, the known effects of gut microbiota on brain function and behaviour alongside the effects of gut microbiota in the pathogenesis of numerous neurological conditions, it is reasonably safe to speculate that Alzheimer's disease may first begin in the gut, and principally relates to an imbalance in gut microbiota (Akbari et al., 2016; Hu et al., 2016).

As Figure 3 illustrates the gut brain axis is an extremely complex bidirectional communication network between the gut and the brain (Dinan and Cryan, 2016). In those who are healthy the gut microbiota is generally stable, forming a symbiotic relationship with the host. However, anything that disrupts or interferes with the relationship may cause dysfunction of the brain, digestive system and metabolism (Cryan and O'Mahony, 2011). In a small number of studies the modulation of gut microbiota correlates with changes in cognitive behaviour. It has been shown that modulation of gut microbiota by probiotics, antibiotic intervention and faecal microbiota transplantation can modulate host cognitive behaviour (Hu et al., 2016). Stress can also influence the composition of gut microbiota, and can compromise the bi-directional communication between the brain and the gut. This in turn may also influence stress reactivity (Foster and Neufeld, 2013). Bhattacharjee and Lukiw (2013) argue that it is remarkable that neuronal signalling pathways along the bidirectional gut–brain axis remain poorly understood despite their obvious importance, in coordinating metabolic and nutritive function and their functional disruption in chronic diseases such as metabolic syndrome, diabetes, obesity, anxiety, autoimmune disease, and stress induced neuropsychiatric diseases.

Oxidative stress, inflammation, and chronic neuro-inflammation are associated with many neurodegenerative disorders of the central nervous system including Alzheimer's disease (Leszek et al., 2016). It has been shown that alterations in micronutrients are a risk factor in Alzheimer's disease (Taghizadeh et al., 2014). The microbiota in the gut are under the influence of genetics, diet, metabolism, age, geography, antibiotic treatment, and stress (Hufeldt et al., 2010), and probiotics (Akbari et al., 2016). Gareau (2014) has shown a clear association between changes in microbiota and cognitive behaviours. Davari et al. (2013) have argued that, within the animal model, an optimal function of the microbiota-gut–brain axis in electrophysiological aspects of the brain action is a necessity. There are however only a small number of studies that have explored the effects of probiotics on improving cognitive disorders (Bhattacharjee and Lukiw, 2013; Davari et al., 2013). Akbari et al. (2016) however have explored the probiotic supplementation on cognitive function and metabolic status in Alzheimer's disease. They explored 60 patients aged between 60 and 95 with Alzheimer's disease, the intervention group (n = 30) received 200 mL/day of probiotic milk containing *Lactobacillus acidophilus*, *Lactobacillus casei*, *Bifidobacterium bifidum*, and *Lactobacillus fermentum* ($2 \times 10_9$ CFU/g for each) for 12 weeks. Patients were tested primarily on the Mini-Mental State Examination (MMSE) used to assess cognition in Alzheimer's disease patients, other tests included biomarkers for oxidative stress information and metabolic profiles. The results appeared to show an improvement in cognitive performance following probiotic administration when compared to controls, but results for biomarkers of oxidative stress and inflammation and other lipid profiles were negligible. However, other biomarkers showed favourable effects for example, high sensitivity C-reactive protein (hs-CRP), markers for insulin metabolism and serum levels of triglycerides and Very Low-Density Lipids (VLDL). The authors of the study argued that probiotic supplementation show some hopeful trends that warrant further study to assess whether probiotics could have a clinically significant impact on cognitive symptoms.

Conclusion

The gut microbiota comprises of a complex community of microorganisms that reside in our gastrointestinal ecosystem, alterations to this complex fragile ecosystem influence not only various gastrointestinal disorders but also central nervous system disorders such as Alzheimer's disease. Alzheimer's disease is one of the most common forms of dementia which is a neurodegenerative disorder associated with impaired cognition. Dementia is one of the most challenging medical problems facing modern societies around the globe, and despite the enormous efforts to combat the condition a medical cure remains elusive. Alzheimer's disease is characterised by extracellular deposits of extracellular amyloid ß, senile plaques and intracellular neurofibrillary tangles. It is also recognised that Alzheimer's disease is an interaction between genetics and environmental factors, with apolipoprotein being one of the most common susceptible genes. There is however growing evidence which suggests that human gut commensal microbiota modulates brain function, and behaviour via the microbiota gut–brain-axis. The small number of studies that have explored this area tend to demonstrate that probiotics can not only affect microbiota but can also influence cognitive behaviour or Alzheimer's related pathogenesis. Work in this area may help advance the discovery of biomarkers that may lead to early diagnosis of Alzheimer's disease and potentially to therapeutic and preventative measures.

References

Akbari E, Asemi Z, Daneshvar Kakhaki R, Bahmani F, Kouchaki E, Tamtaji OR, Hamidi GA and Salami M (2016) Effect of probiotic supplementation on cognitive function and metabolic status in Alzheimer's disease: A randomized, double-blind and controlled trial. Frontiers in Aging Neuroscience 8: 256. doi:10.3389/fnagi.2016.00256.

Alzheimer's Association (2017) 2017 Alzheimer's disease facts and figures. Alzheimer's & Dementia 13: 325–373.

American Psychiatric Association (2013) Diagnostic and Statistical Manual of Mental Disorders, 5th Edition. Arlington: American Psychiatric Publishing.

Bauer KC, Huus KE and Finlay BB (2016) Microbes and the mind: emerging hallmarks of the gut microbiota–brain axis. Cellular Microbiology 18(5): 632–644. doi:10.1111/cmi.12585.

Bhattacharjee S and Lukiw WJ (2013) Alzheimer's disease and the microbiome. Frontiers in Cellular Neuroscience 7: 153. doi:10.3389/fncel.2013.00153 PMCID:PMC3775450.

Biagi E, Candela M, Turroni S, Garagnani P, Franceschi C and Brigidi P (2013) Ageing and gut microbes: perspectives for health maintenance and longevity. Pharmacological Research 69(1): 11–20. doi:0.1111/j.1574-695X.2008.00392.x.

Biasucci G, Rubini M, Riboni S, Morelli L, Bessi E and Retetangos C (2010) Mode of delivery affects the bacterial community in the newborn gut. Early Human Development 86(1): 13–15. doi:10.1016/j.earlhumdev.2010.01.004.

Breslow JL, Zannis VI, SanGiacomo TR, Third J, Tracy T and Glueck CJ (1982) Studies of familial type III hyperlipoproteinemia using as a genetic marker the apoE phenotype E2/2. Journal of Lipid Research 23(8): 1224–1235. PMCID:7175379.

Chapman J, Vinokurov S, Achiron A, Karussis D, Mitosek–Szewczyk K, Birnbaum M, Michaelson DM and Korczyn A (2001) APOE genotype is a major predictor of long-term progression of disability in MS. Neurology 56(3): 312–316. doi:10.1212/WNL.56.3.312.

Claesson MJ, Jeffery IB, Conde S, Power SE, O'Connor EM, Cusack S, Harris HMB, Coakley M, Lakshminarayanan B, O'Sullivan O, Fitzgerald GF, Deane J, O'Connor M, Hardnedy N, O'Connor K, O'Mahony D, VanSinderen D, Wallace M, Brennan L, Stanton C, Marchesi JR, Fitzgerald AP, Shananan F, Hill C, Ross RP and O'Toole PW (2012) Gut microbiota composition correlates with diet and health in the elderly. Nature 488(7410): 178–184. doi:10.1038/nature11319.

Corder E, Saunders A, Strittmatter W, Schmechel D, Gaskell P, Small GA, Roses AD, Haines JL and Pericak-Vance MA (1993) Gene dose of apolipoprotein E type 4 allele and the risk of Alzheimer's disease in late onset families. Science 261(5123): 921–923. doi:10.1126/science.8346443.

Cryan JF and O'Mahony S (2011) The microbiome-gut–brain axis: from bowel to behavior. Neurogastroenterology and Motility 23(3): 187–192. doi:10.1111/j.1365-2982.2010.01664.x.

Cryan JF and Dinan TG (2012) Mind-altering microorganisms: the impact of the gut microbiota on brain and behaviour. Nature Reviews Neuroscience 13(10): 701–712. doi:10.1038/nrn3346.

Davari S, Talaei S and Alaei H (2013) Probiotics treatment improves diabetes-induced impairment of synaptic activity and cognitive function: behavioral and electrophysiological proofs for microbiome–gut–brain axis. Neuroscience 240: 287–296. doi:10.1016/j.neuroscience.2013.02.055.

De Filippo C, Cavalieri D, Di Paola M, Ramazzotti M, Poullet JB, Massart S, Collini S, Pieraccini G and Lionetti P (2010) Impact of diet in shaping gut microbiota revealed by a comparative study in children from Europe and rural Africa. Proceedings of the National Academy of Sciences 107(33): 14691–14696. doi:10.1073/pnas.1005963107.

Deary IJ, Whiteman MC, Pattie A, Starr JM, Hayward C, Wright AF, Carothers A and Whalley LJ (2002) Ageing: Cognitive change and the APOE 4 allele. Nature 418(6901): 932–932. doi:10.1038/418932a.

Dinan TG and Cryan JF (2016) Gut Instincts: microbiota as a key regulator of brain development, ageing and neurodegeneration. The Journal of Physiology. doi:10.1113/JP273106.

Dominguez-Bello MG, Costello EK, Contreras M, Magris M, Hidalgo G, Fierer N and Knight R (2010) Delivery mode shapes the acquisition and structure of the initial microbiota across multiple body habitats in newborns. Proceedings of the National Academy of Sciences 107(26): 11971–11975. doi:10.1073/pnas.1002601107.

Duncan S, Belenguer A, Holtrop G, Johnstone A, Flint H and Lobley G (2007) Reduced dietary intake of carbohydrates by obese subjects results in decreased concentrations of butyrate and butyrate-producing bacteria in feces. Applied and Environmental Microbiology 73(4): 1073–1078. doi:10.1128/AEM.02340-06.

Duncan S and Flint H (2013) Probiotics and prebiotics and health in ageing populations. Maturitas 75(1): 44–50. doi:10.1016/j.maturitas.2013.02.004.

Farlow M, He Y, Tekin S, Xu J, Lane R and Charles H (2004) Impact of APOE in mild cognitive impairment. Neurology 63(10): 1898–1901. doi:10.1212/01.WNL.0000144279.21502.B7.

Finegold SM, Dowd SE, Gontcharova V, Liu C, Henley KE, Wolcott RD, Youn E, Summanen PH, Granpeesheh D, Dixon D, Liu M, Molitoris DR and Green JA 3rd (2010) Pyrosequencing study of fecal microflora of autistic and control children. Anaerobe 16(4): 444–453. doi:10.1016/j.anaerobe.2010.06.008.

Flint HJ (2011) Obesity and the gut microbiota. Journal of Clinical Gastroenterology 45: S128–S132. doi:10.1097/MCG.0b013e31821f44c4.

Foster JA and Neufeld K-AM (2013) Gut–brain axis: how the microbiome influences anxiety and depression. Trends in Neurosciences 36(5): 305–312. doi:10.1016/j.tins.2013.01.005.

Frank DN, Amand ALS, Feldman RA, Boedeker EC, Harpaz N and Pace NR (2007) Molecular-phylogenetic characterization of microbial community imbalances in human inflammatory bowel diseases. Proceedings of the National Academy of Sciences 104(34): 13780–13785. doi:10.1073/pnas.0706625104.

Gareau MG (2014) Microbiota-gut–brain axis and cognitive function. Microbial Endocrinology: The Microbiota-Gut–Brain Axis in Health and Disease (pp. 357–371): Springer.

Ghebranious N, Ivacic L, Mallum J and Dokken C (2005) Detection of ApoE E2, E3 and E4 alleles using MALDI-TOF mass spectrometry and the homogeneous mass-extend technology. Nucleic Acids Research 33(17): e149–e149. doi:10.1093/nar/gni155.

Heavey PM, Savage S-AH, Parrett A, Cecchini C, Edwards CA and Rowland IR (2003) Protein-degradation products and bacterial enzyme activities in faeces of breast-fed and formula-fed infants. British Journal of Nutrition 89(04): 509–515. doi:10.1079/BJN2002814.

Hooper LV and Gordon JI (2001) Commensal host-bacterial relationships in the gut. Science 292(5519): 1115–1118. doi:10.1126/science.1058709.

Hu X, Wang T and Jin F (2016) Alzheimer's disease and gut microbiota. Sci China Life Sci 59(10): 1006–1023. doi:10.1007/s11427-016-5083-9.

Hufeldt MR, Nielsen DS, Vogensen FK, Midtvedt T and Hansen AK (2010) Variation in the gut microbiota of laboratory mice is related to both genetic and environmental factors. Comparative Medicine 60(5): 336–347.

Hurd MD, Martorell P, Delavande A, Mullen KJ and Langa KM (2013) Monetary costs of dementia in the United States. New England Journal of Medicine 368(14): 1326–1334. doi:10.1056/NEJMsa1204629.

Isolauri E (2017) Microbiota and Obesity Intestinal Microbiome: Functional Aspects in Health and Disease. Karger Publishers 88: 95–106.

Jeffery IB, O'Toole PW, Öhman L, Claesson MJ, Deane J, Quigley EM and Simrén M (2012) An irritable bowel syndrome subtype defined by species-specific alterations in faecal microbiota. Gut 61(7): 997–1006. doi:10.1136/gutjnl-2011-301501.

Jiang C, Li G, Huang P, Liu Z and Zhao B (2017) The gut microbiota and Alzheimer's disease. Journal of Alzheimer's Disease 58(1): 1–15. doi:10.3233/JAD-161141.

Katzman R (1976) The prevalence and malignancy of Alzheimer disease: a major killer. Archives of Neurology 33(4): 217–218. doi:10.1001/archneur.1976.00500040001001.

Kleerebezem M and Vaughan EE (2009) Probiotic and gut lactobacilli and bifidobacteria: molecular approaches to study diversity and activity. Annual Review of Microbiology 63: 269–290. doi:10.1146/annurev.micro.091208.073341.

Latypova X and Martin L (2014) 2015: Which new directions for Alzheimer's disease? Frontiers in Cellular Neuroscience 8. doi:10.3389/fncel.2014.00417.

Leszek J, Barreto G, Gasiorowski K, Koutsouraki E and Aliev G (2016) Inflammatory mechanisms and oxidative stress as key factors responsible for progression of neurodegeneration: role of brain innate immune system. CNS & Neurological Disorders-Drug Targets (Formerly Current Drug Targets-CNS & Neurological Disorders) 15(3): 329–336.

Ley RE, Turnbaugh PJ, Klein S and Gordon JI (2006) Microbial ecology: human gut microbes associated with obesity. Nature 444(7122): 1022–1023. doi:10.1038/4441022a.

Li J, Zhao F, Wang Y, Chen J, Tao J, Tian G, Wu S, Liu W, Cui Q, Geng B, Zhang W, Weldon R, Auguste K, Yang L, Liu X, Chen L, Yang X, Zhu B and Cai J (2017) Gut microbiota dysbiosis contributes to the development of hypertension. Microbiome 5(1): 14. doi:10.1186/s40168-016-0222-x.

Mahley RW (1988) Apolipoprotein E: cholesterol transport protein with expanding role in cell biology. Science 240(4852): 622. doi:10.1126/science.3283935.

McKeith I, Mintzer J, Aarsland D, Burn D, Chiu H, Cohen-Mansfield J, Dickson D, Dubois B, Duda JE, Feldman H, Gauthier S, Halliday G, Lawlor B, Lippa C, Lopex OL, Machado JC, O'Brien J, Playfer J and Reid W (2004) Dementia with Lewy bodies. The Lancet Neurology 3(1): 19–28. doi:10.1016/S1474-4422(03)00619-7.

Meurman JH (2010) Oral microbiota and cancer. Journal of Oral Microbiology 2(1): 5195. doi:10.3402/jom.v2i0.5195.

Naseribafrouei A, Hestad K, Avershina E, Sekelja M, Linløkken A, Wilson R and Rudi K (2014) Correlation between the human fecal microbiota and depression. Neurogastroenterology and Motility 26(8): 1155–1162. doi:10.1111/nmo.12378.

O'Brien JT and Thomas A (2015) Vascular dementia. The Lancet 386(10004): 1698–1706. doi:10.1016/S0140-6736(15)00463-8.

O'Toole PW and Claesson MJ (2010) Gut microbiota: Changes throughout the lifespan from infancy to elderly. International Dairy Journal 20(4): 281–291. doi:10.1016/j.idairyj.2009.11.010.

Ouwehand AC, Bergsma N, Parhiala R, Lahtinen S, Gueimonde M, Finne-Soveri H, Strandberg T, Pitakala K and Salminen S (2008) Bifidobacterium microbiota and parameters of immune function in elderly subjects. FEMS Immunology and Medical Microbiology 53(1): 18–25. doi:0.1111/j.1574-695X.2008.00392.x.

Prince M, Bryce R, Albanese E, Wimo A, Ribeiro W and Ferri CP (2013) The global prevalence of dementia: a systematic review and metaanalysis. Alzheimer's & Dementia 9(1): 63–75. e62. doi:10.1016/j.jalz.2012.11.007.

Qin N, Yang F, Li A, Prifti E, Chen Y, Shao L, Guo J, Chatelier EL, Yao J, Wu L, Zhou J, Ni S, Liu L, Pons N, Batto JM, Kennedy SP, Leonard P, Yuan C, Ding W, chen Y, Hu X, Zheng B, Qian G, Xu Wei, Ehrlich SD, Zheng S and Li L (2014) Alterations of the human gut microbiome in liver cirrhosis. Nature 513(7516): 59–64. doi:10.1038/nature13568.

Rabinovici GD and Miller BL (2010) Frontotemporal lobar degeneration. CNS Drugs 24(5): 375–398. doi:10.2165/11533100-000000000-00000.

Reitz C, Brayne C and Mayeux R (2011) Epidemiology of Alzheimer disease. Nature Reviews: Neurology 7(3): 137–152. doi:10.1038/nrneurol.2011.2.

Roberts CL, Keita ÅV, Duncan SH, O'Kennedy N, Söderholm JD, Rhodes JM and Campbell BJ (2010) Translocation of Crohn's disease *Escherichia coli* across M-cells: contrasting effects of soluble plant fibres and emulsifiers. Gut 59(10): 1331–1339. doi:10.1136/gut.2009.195370.

Russell WR, Duncan SH and Flint HJ (2013) The gut microbial metabolome: modulation of cancer risk in obese individuals. Proceedings of the Nutrition Society 72(01): 178–188. doi:10.1017/S0029665112002881.

Sampson TR and Mazmanian SK (2015) Control of brain development, function, and behavior by the microbiome. Cell Host & Microbe 17(5): 565–576. doi:10.1016/j.chom.2015.04.011.

Scheperjans F, Aho V, Pereira PA, Koskinen K, Paulin L, Pekkonen E, Haapaniemi E, Kaakkola S, Eerola-Rautio J, Pohja M, Kinnuunen E, Murros K and Auvinen P (2015) Gut microbiota are related to Parkinson's disease and clinical phenotype. Movement Disorders 30(3): 350–358. doi:10.1002/mds.26069.

Schneider JA, Arvanitakis Z, Bang W and Bennett DA (2007) Mixed brain pathologies account for most dementia cases in community-dwelling older persons. Neurology 69(24): 2197–2204. doi:10.1212/01.wnl.0000271090.28148.24.

Schneider JA, Arvanitakis Z, Leurgans SE and Bennett DA (2009) The neuropathology of probable Alzheimer disease and mild cognitive impairment. Annals of Neurology 66(2): 200–208. doi:10.1002/ana.21706.

Taghizadeh M, Talaei SA, Djazayeri A and Salami M (2014) Vitamin D supplementation restores suppressed synaptic plasticity in Alzheimer's disease. Nutritional Neuroscience 17(4): 172–177. doi:10.1179/1476830513Y.0000000080.

Tilg H and Moschen AR (2014) Microbiota and diabetes: an evolving relationship. Gut 63(9): 1513–1521. doi:10.1136/gutjnl-2014-306928.

Tilg H, Grander C and Moschen AR (2016) How does the microbiome affect liver disease? Clinical Liver Disease 8(5): 123–126. doi:10.1002/cld.586.

Toward R, Montandon S, Walton G and Gibson GR (2012) Effect of prebiotics on the human gut microbiota of elderly persons. Gut Microbes 3(1): 57–60. doi:10.4161/gmic.19411.

Tremlett H, Bauer KC, Appel-Cresswell S, Finlay BB and Waubant E (2017) The gut microbiome in human neurological disease: A review. Annals of Neurology 81(3): 369–382. doi:10.1002/ana.24901.

Viswanathan A, Rocca WA and Tzourio C (2009) Vascular risk factors and dementia How to move forward? Neurology 72(4): 368–374. doi:10.1212/01.wnl.0000341271.90478.8e.

Woodmansey EJ (2007) Intestinal bacteria and ageing. Journal of Applied Microbiology 102(5): 1178–1186. doi:10.1111/j.1365-2672.2007.03400.x.

World Health Organization (2016) World Health Statistics 2016: Monitoring Health for the SDGs Sustainable Development Goals: World Health Organization.

CHAPTER 13

Probiotics and Autistic Spectrum Disorder

Derek Larkin[1,]* and *Colin R Martin*[2]

INTRODUCTION

Autistic spectrum disorder is a serious developmental disorder with increasing prevalence, said to affect 14.6 per 1,000 (one in 68) children aged 8 years (Christensen, 2016). Autistic spectrum disorder is characterised by a spectrum of symptoms which includes decreased verbal skills, social withdrawal, repetitive behaviour, insistence to retain an unusual response to sensory stimuli (Critchfield et al., 2011). Autism was first identified by an American psychiatrist named Theo Kanner, in a paper published in 1943 entitled 'Autistic disturbances of affective contact' (Kanner, 1943). A short time later Hans Asperger published a paper entitled 'Autistic psychopathy in children' (Asperger, 1944). Even though both papers describe individuals with different underlying behavioural traits, there are however undeniable similarities (see Figure 1).

Autistic spectrum disorders are a diverse group of complex, persistent and pervasive neurodevelopmental conditions which are characterized by impairments in social communication, social interaction, often restrictive and repetitive patterns of behaviour, interests or activities (American Psychiatric Association, 2013; Masi et al., 2017). Impairments range from mild to profound in which all aspects of daily functioning and quality of life are affected (de Vries and Geurts, 2015; Perry et al., 2009). Current treatments include specialised behavioural interventions (Seida et al., 2009) and pharmacological interventions which assist in comorbid or associated symptoms (Leskovec et al., 2008) including mental health, for example anxiety,

[1] Edge Hill University, St Helens Road, Ormsirk, Lancashire, L39 4QP.
[2] Faculty of Society and Health, Buckinghamshire New University, Uxbridge Campus, 106 Oxford Road, Uxbridge, Middlesex, UB8 1NA, UK.
* Corresponding author

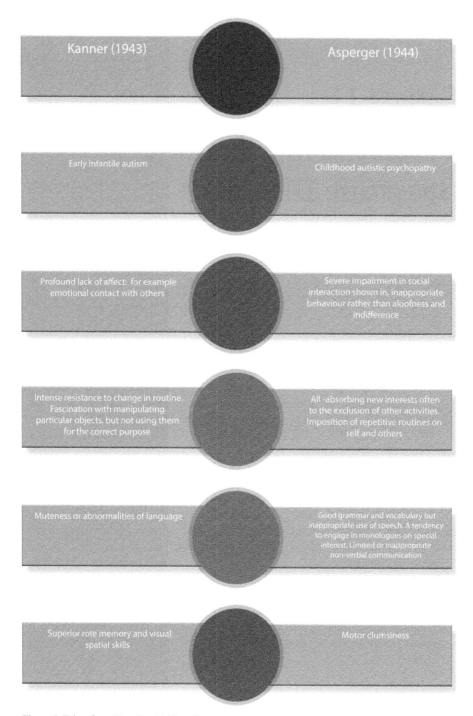

Figure 1 Taken from (Boucher, 2008, p. 5).

depression and attention deficit/hyperactivity disorder (Matson and Shoemaker, 2009; Simonoff et al., 2008). Autistic spectrum disorder is a heterogeneous condition with a complex and incomplete etiology. The causes of autistic spectrum disorders are currently the focus of intense study with particular focus on environment, genetics and epigenetic factors. Also under intense investigation is the understanding that a prominent subgroup of individuals with autistic spectrum disorder suffer from gastrointestinal dysfunction, the cause of which is presently unknown. Activation of the mucosal immune response, in the presence of abnormal gut microbiota have been observed in children with autistic spectrum disorders. Often associated conditions include irritability, tantrums, aggression and sleep disturbances. Modulating the gut bacteria with short term antibiotic treatments has been known to temporarily improve behavioral symptoms. Probiotics have been shown to influence microbiota composition, therefore may be a useful novel therapeutic tool to restore normal gut microbiota, reduce inflammation and ameliorate behavioral symptoms associated with autistic spectrum disorders (Critchfield et al., 2011; Masi et al., 2017).

Autistic Spectrum Disorder

Autistic Spectrum disorder, sometimes referred to as disorder(s) as a reflection of the complex etiology, is a developmental neuropsychiatric syndrome with onset before the age of 3 years (Geschwind, 2011). The conceptualization of autistic spectrum disorder is based on the initial observations of Kanner (1943) in which he described 11 children with autism, mainly boys, with a combination of severe language and social dysfunction, in the presence of repetitive restricted behaviors. Since Kanner (1943) and Asperger (1944) autistic spectrum disorder has come to represent a quantitative spectrum of impairments, as opposed to a discrete disorder (Constantino and Todd, 2003; Wing, 1988). The move from 'Autism' to 'Autistic spectrum disorder(s)' is an attempt to crystallize the notion that patients represent a variable population, who suffer from clinically representative major cognitive and behavioral disruptions, as opposed to a distinct clinical disorder (Geschwind, 2011). This division also represents the underlying spectrum of etiologies thought to be involved in this condition.

The diagnosis for autistic spectrum disorder is not based on aetiology, but on expert observation and assessment of behaviour cognition (Geschwind, 2011). In the DSM-V (American Psychiatric Association, 2013 outlined in Tables 1 and 2) Asperger syndrome has been removed and the diagnostic criteria for autism and has been modified to autistic spectrum disorder.

Autistic Spectrum Disorders: an Historical Perspective

Studies conducted in the 1960s and 1970s defined autism as a severe condition usually accompanied by intellectual disability (Gillberg and Wing, 1999). Autism was recognised as a unique clinical diagnosis by the DSM-III in 1980 (American Psychiatric Association, 1980), which provided a diagnostic criterion for infantile autism and pervasive developmental disorders. As described previously autism has become recognised as a spectrum disorder of behavioural characteristics which

Table 1 Taken from the DSM-5 (American Psychiatric Association, 2013, pp. 50–52) and Carpenter (2013).

DSM-5 Autism Spectrum Disorder

A. Persistent deficit in social communication and social interaction across multiple context, as manifested by the following, currently or by history.
 	
   A1. Deficits in social-emotional reciprocity; ranging from abnormal social approach and failure of normal back and forth conversation through reduced sharing of interests, emotions, and affect and response to total lack of initiation of social interaction.
     • Abnormal social approach
     • Failure of normal back and forth conversation
     • Reduced sharing of interests
     • Reduced sharing of emotional/affect
     • Lack of initiation of social interactions
     • Poor social imitation

A2. Deficits in nonverbal communicative behaviours used for social interaction; ranging from poorly integrated-verbal and nonverbal communication, through abnormalities in eye contact and body-language, or deficits in understanding and use of nonverbal communication, to total lack of facial expression or gestures.
     • Impairments social use of eye contact
     • Poor understanding of body posture of both self and others
     • Poor understanding of non-verbal gestures—for example pointing or waving

A3. Deficits in developing and maintaining relationships appropriate to developmental level (beyond those with caregivers); ranging from difficulties adjusting behaviour to suit different social contexts through difficulties in sharing imaginative play and in making friends to an apparent absence of interest in people.
     • Deficit in developing and maintaining relationships appropriate to developmental level
     • Difficulty adjusting behaviour to suit social context
     • Difficulties and sharing imaginative play
     • Difficulties in making friends
     • Absence of interest in others

B. Restrictive, repetitive pattern of behaviour, interests or activities as manifested by at least two of the following, currently or by history.
 	
   B1. Stereotyped or repetitive speech, motor movements, or use of objects (such as simple motor stereotypes, echolalia, repetitive use of objects, or idiosyncratic phrases).
     • Stereotyped repetitive speech, e.g., pedantic or unusually formal language, idiosyncratic or metaphorical language.
     • Stereotyped repetitive motor movements, e.g., repetitive hand movements such as clapping, finger flicking, flapping or twisting. Stereotyped or complex whole-body movement, such as swaying or spinning.
     • Stereotyped repetitive use of objects, e.g., non-functional play with objects, repetitive lining up of toys or objects.

B2. Excessive adherence to routines, ritualized patterns of verbal or nonverbal behaviour, or excessive resistance to change (such as motoric rituals, insistence on same route or food, repetitive questioning, or extreme distress at small changes).
     • Adherence to routine, e.g., insistence on rigidity following specific routines—in relation to food, bed time, etc.
     • Unusual routine
     • Ritualised patterns of verbal and non-verbal
     • Excesses resistance to change
     • Rigid thinking

Table 1 contd. ...

... Table 1 contd.

DSM-5 Autism Spectrum Disorder
B3. Highly restricted, fixated interests that is abnormal in intensity or focus (such as strong attachment to or preoccupation with unusual objects, excessively circumscribed or perseverative interests). • Preoccupations and obsessions • Interests that are abnormal in intensity • Narrow range of interests • Overly perfectionists • Preoccupation (colour; timetables; historical events)
B4. Hyper- or hypo-reactivity to sensory input or unusual interest in sensory aspects of environment (such as apparent indifference to pain/heat/cold, adverse response to specific sounds or textures, excessive smelling or touching of objects, fascination with lights or spinning objects). • Unusually high tolerance for pain • Preoccupation with texture touch • Unusual visual exploration/activity, e.g., close visual inspection of objects • In all domains of sensory stimuli—auditory, olfactory, taste, vestibular and visual, e.g., unusual responses to sensory input—becoming distressed by atypical sounds • Unusual sensory exploration of objects, e.g., licking or sniffing objects
C. Symptoms must be present in early childhood but may not become fully manifest antisocial demands exceed limited capacities
D. Symptoms together limit and impair everyday functioning

involve varying degrees of functional limitations. The DSM IV (American Psychiatric Association, 2000) introduced a revised diagnostic criteria, with five subtypes of autism, (1) Autistic disorder (2) Asperger syndrome (3) pervasive developmental disorder-not otherwise specified (PDD-NOS) (4) Childhood disintegrative disorder (5) Retts disorder. Autistic disorder, Asperger syndrome and pervasive developmental disorder—not otherwise specified comprise Autistic spectrum disorder (Christensen, 2016). The most recent edition of the DSM (American Psychiatric Association, 2013) edition 5, redefined autistic spectrum disorder into a single entity alongside, a number of changes in diagnostic classification (see Tables 1 and 2).

Probiotics

The word "Probiotics" means "for life" and is currently used to describe a group of bacteria that when administered in sufficient quantities is able to confer beneficial effects on human and animal host (Bedaiwi and Inman, 2014). The interest in probiotics has grown exponentially during the past several years and has penetrated many cultures due to the functional properties associated with improved health. It has been argued that probiotics improve human health through varying modes of action, principally restoration of host microbiota, re-establishing the intestinal barrier function, inducing a state of homoeostasis in the immune system, support of digestive functioning and by providing several trace nutrient elements to the host (Etzold et al., 2014). Worldwide research has aimed to determine innovative approaches in

Table 2 Taken from DSM-5 (American Psychiatric Association, 2013, p. 52).

Severity Levels for Autistic Spectrum Disorder		
Severity Level for autistic spectrum disorder	Social communication	Restricted interests and repetitive behaviours
Level 3 'Requiring very substantial support'	Severe deficits in verbal and nonverbal social communication skills cause severe impairments in functioning; very limited initiation of social interactions and minimal response to social overtures from others.	Inflexibility of behaviour, extreme difficulty coping with change or other restricted/ repetitive behaviours markedly interfere with functioning in all spheres.
Level 2 'Requiring substantial support'	Marked deficits in verbal and nonverbal social communication skills; social impairments apparent even with supports in place; limited initiation of social interactions and reduced or abnormal response to social overtures from others.	Inflexibility of behaviour, difficulty coping with change, or other restrict/repetitive behaviours appear frequently enough to be obvious to casual observer and interfere with functioning in a variety of contexts.
Level 1 'Requiring support'	Without supports in place, deficits in social communication cause noticeable impairments. Has difficulty initiating social interactions and demonstrates clear examples of atypical or unsuccessful responses to social overtures of others. May appear to have decreased interest in social interactions.	Inflexibility of behaviour causes significant interference with function in one or more context. Difficulty switching between activities. Problems of organisation and planning hamper independence.

the field of clinical health using probiotic formulation. There is growing scientific and commercial interest in probiotics in relation to public health. Ongoing research has generated numerous new and interesting working hypotheses in relation to manipulating gut bacteria to maintain and restore health. The connection between gut microbiota, intestinal disease and autism is a potential area for research. Recent research has investigated the link between gut microbiota and autistic spectrum disorder in an animal model, they found that autistic spectrum disorders may be elicited by microbes and its associated metabolic compositional and structural shifts (Hsiao et al., 2013). This group of researchers also found the administration of the probiotic *Bacteroides fragilis*, relieved symptoms thus demonstrating the potential for a therapeutic strategy for neurodevelopment disorders such as Autistic spectrum disorder.

Probiotics and Autistic Spectrum Disorder

Studies conducted over the last few decades have increasingly revealed the central role of the gut microbiota in postnatal development and maturation of immune and endocrine systems in the development of disease states. Dysbiosis (the state of unbalance and disrupted microbiota communities), has been shown to play a significant role in the aetiology and pathogenesis of numerous medical conditions including autoimmune diseases, such as rheumatoid arthritis, type I diabetes, and inflammatory bowel disease, and has also been implicated in psychopathologies, such as depression and anxiety. Other conditions such as necrotising enterocolitis in infants, systemic infection following cancer chemotherapy, dental caries, and obesity have also been implicated in the balance and disruption of microbial communities (Ding et al., 2017; Hooper et al., 2012; Penders et al., 2007; Taur et al., 2012). There is now increasing evidence to suggest a brain–gut–microbe connection, with dysbiosis and autistic spectrum disorder.

Under normal circumstances the human body share a symbiotic relationship with a large number of bacteria and microorganisms (with the exception of the very young and very old, and those suffering from particular disease states). The number and variety of bacteria and microorganisms is far greater than we had previously comprehended (Eckburg et al., 2005). Studies have also concluded that under normal circumstances intestinal microbiota are largely comprised of anaerobic bacteria which are non-pathogenic and serve a variety of functions that are beneficial to the host (Ding et al., 2017). These bacteria are generally responsible for absorbing nutrients and the production of short chain fatty acids, vitamins and amino acid synthesis from ammonia and urea, they are also involved in the detoxification of xenobiotics, and play a part in host immunity, and unknown to prevent the overproduction of pathogenic bacteria, and maintain colonic wall health (Ding et al., 2017; Hooper et al., 2012; Sekirov et al., 2010). Evidence suggests the commensal organisms live exclusively within the human intestinal system, and nowhere else, this therefore suggests an historical relationship that stretches back in our evolutionary past, the clinical implications of this realisation has yet to be discovered (Ding et al., 2017). The prevalence of gastrointestinal symptoms in autistic spectrum disorder has a number of common symptoms, including diarrhoea, constipation, vomiting and reflux, abdominal pain and discomfort, gassiness and unusual foul smelling faeces (Critchfield et al., 2011; Li et al., 2017), these symptoms are very similar to those of irritable bowel syndrome (Buie et al., 2010). Studies have reported altered gastrointestinal motility and increased intestinal permeability (de Magistris et al., 2010). Whereas other studies have found a high prevalence of inflammatory bowel disease, and other gastrointestinal disorders in patients with autistic spectrum disorder (Kohane et al., 2012). The prevalence of gastrointestinal symptoms in children with autistic spectrum disorder is not entirely clear however it has been estimated to affect 9 to 70% of individuals (Buie et al., 2010). This wide range of difference may be a combination of a number of effects including differences in study populations and the definition of gastrointestinal symptomology, what is however not in dispute is that gastrointestinal symptoms are significant problems in individuals with autistic spectrum disorder, and indeed may be an important contributor to behavioural difficulties (Buie et al., 2010; Ding et al., 2017).

Studies have shown that individuals with autistic spectrum disorder who also have gastrointestinal symptomology appeared to display higher rates of irritability, anxiety and social withdrawal, compared to individuals with autistic spectrum disorder but without the gastrointestinal symptoms (Nikolov et al., 2009). Buie et al. (2010) argues that self-injurious behaviour, aggression, and sleep disturbances alongside irritability may be behavioural manifestations of abdominal pain, and gastrointestinal disquiet in individuals with autistic spectrum disorder. Adams et al. (2011) have shown a significant correlation between gastrointestinal dysfunction and severity of autistic spectrum disorder behaviours, across domains such as speech, social interaction, and general behaviour. The proviso to all of these studies is that they do not attribute cause and effect but they do seem to indicate the importance of exploring gastrointestinal symptoms in children with autism, with the goal of alleviating gastrointestinal symptoms within this vulnerable population (Ding et al., 2017). It could be argued that gastrointestinal symptomology in autistic spectrum disorder do not share a causal relationship, however, it could equally be argued that the gastrointestinal symptoms indicate that the gut may play a pivotal role in the aetiology of autistic spectrum disorder at least within a subset of patients (Ding et al., 2017).

There has been an observation that behavioural symptoms and chronic diarrhoea appear after repeated courses of antibiotics in a subset of children with autistic spectrum disorder. The cause of these gastrointestinal symptoms is thought to be a species of toxin producing *Clostridium*. In the faeces of children with autistic spectrum disorder versus healthy controls, a tenfold increase in the levels of *Clostridium* species was reported, alongside a greater diversity of *Clostridium* species (Finegold et al., 2002). The disadvantage with this study is that no comparison was made with autistic spectrum disorder patients without gastrointestinal symptoms, therefore cause and effect cannot be made. Song et al. (2004) reported that there were elevations in three different *Clostridium* groups, *Clostridium bolteae* and *Clostridium* clusters I and XI, in individuals with autistic spectrum disorder however this study did not report the frequency of gastrointestinal symptoms in the subjects (Critchfield et al., 2011). A subsequent study conducted by Parracho et al. (2005) showed that the *Clostridium histolyticum* group which is a known toxin producer (Hatheway, 1990) was elevated in autistic spectrum disorder children compared to healthy unrelated controls but not compared to healthy siblings. The study also concluded that *Clostridium* correlated with gastrointestinal symptoms. Finegold et al. (2010) conducted a pyrosequencing-based study and found numerous differences in faecal microbiota composition among children with autistic spectrum disorder, compared with controls. Amongst the changes observed were shifts at the phylum level towards a higher proportion of *Bacteroidetes* and lower levels of *Firmicutes* in individuals with autistic spectrum disorder. *Bifidobacterium* was found in much lower numbers in those with autistic spectrum disorder whereas *Desulfovibrio* were found in much greater numbers. Curiously the sibling control group had a microbiota composition nearer to that of their autistic spectrum disorder siblings, possibly due to transfer of microbial species within family members, rather than as a consequence of autistic spectrum disorder pathology (Critchfield et al., 2011).

From these studies, the '*Clostridium* hypothesis', the idea that gut microbial imbalance, in the presence of toxin producing *Clostridium* species could contribute to autistic spectrum disorder behavioural symptoms has emerged. The rationale for this hypothesis is based on similarities with known behaviours of other *Clostridium* species that caused toxin mediated disease (Ding et al., 2017). In a small study conducted by Sandler et al. (2000), 11 children with chronic diarrhoea and late onset phenotype of autistic spectrum disorder, were treated for eight weeks with oral vancomycin, an antibiotic used to treat chronic *Clostridium* difficile diarrhoea. Significant improvements in neurobehavioral symptoms (even among individuals scoring within neuro-typical range) were observed in eight of the children, along with improvements in gastrointestinal symptoms. However, these gains in behaviour were temporary, and deteriorated in most cases after termination of the antibiotic treatment. Composition of faecal flora were not reported, neither were gastrointestinal symptomology, the design also suffered from a lack of a control group. The oral administration of vancomycin meant that the antibiotic affect was confined to the intestinal tract and not systematically absorbed; *Clostridium* may have converted into spore-form, which are known to be highly resistant to antibiotics and may have germinated into vegetative effective form, therefore explaining the return of the gastrointestinal symptoms, following the suspension of antibiotic treatment. The findings suggest that the use of antibiotics may target intestinal microbiota that are implicated in neurobehavioral and gastrointestinal symptomology associated with autistic spectrum disorder. Even though further studies support the *Clostridium* hypothesis the precise species responsible has not been determined (Ding et al., 2017). Finegold et al. (2010) report a ten-fold difference in the level of *Clostridium* faeces in children with autistic spectrum disorder with gastrointestinal symptomology, in comparison to healthy control, they also noted a lack of anaerobic bacteria in autistic children. Song et al. (2004) found a higher level of *Clostridium bolteae* in autistic spectrum disorder children whereas Parracho et al. (2005) found high levels of *Clostridium histolyticum*. These results seem to paint a compelling picture of a unique pattern of microflora in children with autistic spectrum disorder with gastrointestinal symptomology.

Other species of gut bacteria have been associated with disturbances in intestinal microbiota, within an autistic spectrum disorder population. *Sutterella* (Williams et al., 2011) is reported at a higher prevalence in individuals with autistic spectrum disorder and gastrointestinal symptomology. Along with *Sutterella* Wang et al. (2013) found high levels of *Ruminococcus torques* in the guts of children with autistic spectrum disorder. *Akkermansia muciniphilia* (De Angelis et al., 2013; Kang et al., 2013), *Desulfovibri* (Finegold et al., 2010) and *Faecalibacterium prausnitzii* (De Angelis et al., 2013) were found in increased abundance, in autistic spectrum disorder children. Kang et al. (2013) found low levels of *Prevotella*. *Prevotella* is associated with good gastrointestinal health. However, because research protocols differ between research laboratories conflicting findings are often reported, nevertheless there appears to be a body of evidence which contests that dysbiosis may be implicated at some level in autistic spectrum disorder. One mechanism for dysbiosis maybe the use of antibiotics, which disrupts normal microbiota health. Another mechanism was proposed by Williams et al. (2011) in which they suggest that defective dissaccharidase and hexose transporter leads to a compromised carbohydrate environment in the distal cecum/ileum, this then may lead to dysbiosis, as the bacteria have an additional substrate in which to colonise (Ding et al., 2017).

Leaky Gut

Under normal circumstances, in a healthy subject the epithelial gut barrier is maintained by tight junctions that control the flow of molecules between the gastrointestinal tract and bloodstream (Ding et al., 2017; Hollander, 1999). Gut microbiota are integral in maintaining cell to cell junctions critical to barrier integrity (Hsiao et al., 2013). When the integrity of the barrier has been compromised this has been termed as a 'leaky gut' which has been linked to a wide range of intestinal systemic disorders (Fasano, 2012). Once the gut becomes leaky it is therefore possible to increase intestinal permeability which may allow the passage of bacteria, toxins and other metabolites which may lead to immune activation (Ding et al., 2017).

Immune Dysfunction

For many years theories have been developed which implicate the possible role of immune dysfunction in autistic spectrum disorder. Even though the studies have been criticised as being underpowered and sometimes conflicting, due to small sample sizes, heterogeneous patient populations and lack of adequate controls (Stigler et al., 2009), many studies have reported abnormal immune activity in a subset of individuals with autistic spectrum disorder. Research has shown abnormal ratios of $CD4^+$ to $CD8^+$, T-cells, T-helper cells—$T_H1/T_H2/T_H17$, cytokine profiles, elevated blood monocytes, decrease lymphocytes, self-activated antibodies to the brain, CNS proteins, neuro-inflammation, imbalance of serums and mucosal, immunoglobulin levels and increase in nitric oxide mechanisms (Ashwood and Wakefield, 2006; Careaga et al., 2010; Critchfield et al., 2011; Enstrom et al., 2009).

The vast majority of the immune system is concentrated in and around the intestinal mucosa; the intestinal microbiota are involved in maturation of the immune system, and are involved in the regulation and function of the immune system (Delcenserie et al., 2008; Hooper and Gordon, 2001). Evidence suggests that probiotics are able to modulate immune system response, dependent upon specific species and strains (Gill and Prasad, 2008; Hooper and Gordon, 2001). Hatakka et al. (2003) reports that the autoimmune response found in rheumatoid arthritis responded well to administration of probiotics, even though there was no statistical difference between experimental groups there were subjected to measures of improvement in symptoms. Limited evidence suggests that probiotics have good *in vivo* capacities to reduce anti-inflammatory cytokines, however their effect on systemic cytokine profiles remain to be proven and may be dependent on microbiota mix *in situ* (Critchfield et al., 2011).

It has been noted by numerous experimental studies that there is a bi-directional communication between the gut, the immune system, and the brain. When individuals are psychologically stressed it can induce dramatic changes in gastrointestinal microbiota in both the human and animal models. Intestinal bacteria are capable of communicating with the central nervous system directly via the vagal sensory nerve fibres and peripheral immune system (Goehler et al., 2007). It has been suggested that gut–brain interactions may contribute to abnormal neural development and therefore may express abnormal behaviours in the host. It has been also suggested that a leaky gut may allow for partially digestive foods and bacterial components to pass into the bloodstream and therefore may interfere directly or indirectly with the central nervous system. A leaky gut may also allow entry for lipopolysaccharides, potent pro-inflammatory compounds of the cell walls of ground negative bacteria. This then may trigger peripheral inflammatory responses that may lead to *de novo* the production of cytokines in the brain (Critchfield et al., 2011). By preventing the weakening of the epithelial barrier, this could limit the possibility of bacterial traffic and their by-products leaking from the gut and causing an inflammatory response.

Administration of probiotics has been known to influence neuronal functioning, and attenuate pro-inflammatory immune responses. Pro-inflammatory immune response has been attenuated by the administration of *Bifidobacteria*. Evidence supports the contention that intestinal dysbiosis or gastrointestinal dysfunction can profoundly affect multiple aspects of mood and cognitive function (Jackson et al., 2015). Both Rao et al. (2009) and Sullivan et al. (2009) found probiotic supplementation may have a beneficial effect on mood related symptoms associated with chronic fatigue syndrome, which is an argument much in line with Logan et al. (2003) who suggested that altered intestinal microbiota contributes to the pathogenesis of chronic fatigue syndrome, and that therapeutic rebalance or modification of intestinal microbiota may have the potential to reduce the symptoms. Studies also appear to show that the administration of specific strains of probiotic can ameliorate some of the symptoms in numerous psychopathologies, including depression, obsessive-compulsive disorder, schizophrenia, and even Alzheimer's disease. Autistic spectrum disorder is just one of numerous disorders that appear to have a complex interplay between genetics and environmental components. There is a range of indications that alterations in intestinal microbiota in the gut might contribute to these disorders in a substantial number of individuals. With specific reference to autistic spectrum disorder probiotics can be used to restore microbiota balance within the intestine, which has been shown to relieve gastrointestinal symptomology and attenuate immunological abnormalities. Additional research needs to be conducted to investigate whether the administration of probiotics directly and measurably affects the behaviour of individuals with autistic spectrum disorder, furthermore additional research needs to be conducted exploring particular specific strains of probiotic, and the potential benefits to the hosts' behaviour and immune response.

Conclusion

Children with autistic spectrum disorder are commonly affected by gastrointestinal symptomology, which may include abdominal pains, constipation and diarrhoea. Over the past few decades there has been growing interest in the use of probiotics in individuals with autistic spectrum disorder to help improve bowel habits, behavioural and social functioning. The influence of the enteric microbiota on the human body has only started to be revealed. Its role in the immune response metabolism and neurological functioning is starting to be elucidated. Dysbiosis is associated with a number of conditions which include inflammatory bowel disease, irritable bowel syndrome, and autism. Probiotics are hypothesised to positively impact gut microbial communities which appeared to affect specific potentially harmful metabolites in children with autistic spectrum disorder. There appears to be increasing body of evidence which demonstrates the clinical of metabolites inhabiting the intestinal tract, and increasing evidence linking dysbiosis and numerous disease states. In individuals with autistic spectrum disorder there appears to be a unique subset of individuals whose health, both physical and mental is reliant on the health and well-being of intestinal microbiota. However, in relation to the direction of causality it is not entirely clear whether dysbiosis is secondary to altered neural-regulation of key intestinal functioning, or whether it has a primary impact on brain development and function.

References

Adams JB, Johansen LJ, Powell LD, Quig D and Rubin RA (2011) Gastrointestinal flora and gastrointestinal status in children with autism–comparisons to typical children and correlation with autism severity. BMC Gastroenterology 11(1): 22. doi:10.1186/1471-230X-11-22.

American Psychiatric Association (1980) Diagnostic and Statistical Manual of Mental Disorders, 3rd Edition. Washington, DC: American Psychiatric Publishing.

American Psychiatric Association (2000) Diagnostic and Statistical Manual of Mental Disorders, 4th Edition, Text Revised (DSM-IV-TR). Washington, DC: American Psychiatric Publishing.

American Psychiatric Association (2013) Diagnostic and Statistical Manual of Mental Disorders, 5th Edition. Washington, DC: American Psychiatric Publishing.

Ashwood P and Wakefield AJ (2006) Immune activation of peripheral blood and mucosal CD3+ lymphocyte cytokine profiles in children with autism and gastrointestinal symptoms. Journal of Neuroimmunology 173(1): 126–134. doi:10.1016/j.jneuroim.2005.12.007.

Asperger H (1944) Die "Autistischen Psychopathen" im Kindesalter. European Archives of Psychiatry and Clinical Neuroscience 117(1): 76–136.

Bedaiwi MK and Inman RD (2014) Microbiome and probiotics: link to arthritis. Current Opinion in Rheumatology 26(4): 410–415. doi:10.1097/BOR.0000000000000075.

Boucher J (2008) The autistic spectrum: Characteristics, causes and practical issues. Sage.

Buie T, Campbell DB, Fuchs GJ, Furuta GT, Levy J, Vande Water J, Whitaker AH, Atkins D, Bauman ML, Beaudet AL, Carr G, Gershon MD, Hyman SL, Jirapinyo P, Jyonouchi H, Kooros K, Kushak R, Levitt P, Levy SE, Lewis JD, Murray Kf, Natowicz MR, Sabra A, Wershil BK, Weston SC, Zeltzer L and Winter H (2010) Evaluation, diagnosis, and treatment of gastrointestinal disorders in individuals with ASDs: a consensus report. Pediatrics 125(Supplement 1): S1–S18.

Careaga M, Van de Water J and Ashwood P (2010) Immune dysfunction in autism: a pathway to treatment. Neurotherapeutics 7(3): 283–292. doi:0.1016/j.nurt.2010.05.003.

Carpenter L (2013) DSM-5 Autistic spectrum disorder: guidelines and criteria exemplars. Retrieved from https://depts.washington.edu/dbpeds/ScreeningTools/DSM-5%28ASD.Guidelines%29Feb2013.pdf.

Christensen DL (2016) Prevalence and characteristics of autism spectrum disorder among children aged 8 years—autism and developmental disabilities monitoring network, 11 sites, United States, 2012. MMWR. Surveillance Summaries 65(3).

Constantino JN and Todd RD (2003) Autistic traits in the general population: a twin study. Archives of General Psychiatry 60(5): 524–530. doi:10.1001/archpsyc.60.5.524.

Critchfield JW, Van Hemert S, Ash M, Mulder L and Ashwood P (2011) The potential role of probiotics in the management of childhood autism spectrum disorders. Gastroenterology Research and Practice, 2011. doi:10.1155/2011/161358.

De Angelis M, Piccolo M, Vannini L, Siragusa S, De Giacomo A, Serrazzanetti DI, Cristofori F, Guerzoni ME, Gobbetti M and Francavilla R (2013) Fecal microbiota and metabolome of children with autism and pervasive developmental disorder not otherwise specified. PloS One 8(10): e76993. doi:10.1371/journal.pone.0076993.

de Magistris L, Familiari V, Pascotto A, Sapone A, Frolli A, Iardino P, Riegler G, Militerni R and Baravaccio C (2010) Alterations of the intestinal barrier in patients with autism spectrum disorders and in their first-degree relatives. Journal of Pediatric Gastroenterology and Nutrition 51(4): 418–424. doi:10.1097/MPG.0b013e3181dcc4a5.

de Vries M and Geurts H (2015) Influence of autism traits and executive functioning on quality of life in children with an autism spectrum disorder. Journal of Autism and Developmental Disorders 45(9): 2734–2743. doi:10.1007/s10803-015-2438-1.

Delcenserie V, Martel D, Lamoureux M, Amiot J, Boutin Y and Roy D (2008) Immunomodulatory effects of probiotics in the intestinal tract. Current Issues in Molecular Biology 10(1/2): 37.

Ding HT, Taur Y and Walkup JT (2017) Gut microbiota and autism: key concepts and findings. Journal of Autism and Developmental Disorders 47(2): 480–489. doi:10.1007/s10803-016-2960-9.

Eckburg PB, Bik EM, Bernstein CN, Purdom E, Dethlefsen L, Sargent M, Gill SR, Nelson KE and Relman DA (2005) Diversity of the human intestinal microbial flora. Science 308(5728): 1635–1638. doi:10.1126/science.1110591.

Enstrom A, Krakowiak P, Onore C, Pessah IN, Hertz-Picciotto I, Hansen RL, Van de Water JA and Ashwood P (2009) Increased IgG4 levels in children with autism disorder. Brain, Behavior, and Immunity 23(3): 389–395. doi:0.1016/j.bbi.2008.12.005.

Etzold S, Kober OI, MacKenzie DA, Tailford LE, Gunning AP, Walshaw J, Hemmings AM and Juge N (2014) Structural basis for adaptation of lactobacilli to gastrointestinal mucus. Environmental Microbiology 16(3): 888–903. doi:10.1111/1462-2920.1237.

Fasano A (2012) Leaky gut and autoimmune diseases. Clinical Reviews in Allergy & Immunology 42(1): 71–78. doi:10.1007/s12016-011-8291-x.

Finegold SM, Molitoris D, Song Y, Liu C, Vaisanen M-L, Bolte E, McTeague M, Sandler R, Wexler H, Marlowe EM, Collins MD, Lawson PA, Summanen P, Baysallar M, Tomzynski TJ, Read E, Johnson E, Rolfe R, Nasir P, Shah H, Haake DA, Manning P and Kaul A (2002) Gastrointestinal microflora studies in late-onset autism. Clinical Infectious Diseases 35(Supplement 1): S6–S16. doi:10.1086/341914.

Finegold SM, Dowd SE, Gontcharova V, Liu C, Henley KE, Wolcott RD, Youn E, Summanen PH, Granpeesheh D, Dixon D, Liu M, Molitoris DR and Green JA 3rd (2010) Pyrosequencing study of fecal microflora of autistic and control children. Anaerobe 16(4): 444–453. doi:10.1016/j.anaerobe.2010.06.008.

Geschwind DH (2011) Genetics of autism spectrum disorders. Trends in Cognitive Sciences 15(9): 409–416. doi:10.1016/j.tics.2011.07.003.

Gill H and Prasad J (2008) Probiotics, immunomodulation, and health benefits. Bioactive Components of Milk (pp. 423–454): Springer.

Gillberg C and Wing L (1999) Autism: not an extremely rare disorder. Acta Psychiatrica Scandinavica 99(6): 399–406. doi:10.1111/j.1600-0447.1999.tb00984.x.

Goehler LE, Lyte M and Gaykema RP (2007) Infection-induced viscerosensory signals from the gut enhance anxiety: implications for psychoneuroimmunology. Brain, Behavior, and Immunity 21(6): 721–726. doi:10.1016/j.bbi.2007.02.005.

Hatakka K, Martio J, Korpela M, Herranen M, Poussa T, Laasanen T, Saxelin M, Vapaatalo H, Moilanen E and Korpela R (2003) Effects of probiotic therapy on the activity and activation of mild rheumatoid arthritis—a pilot study. Scandinavian Journal of Rheumatology 32(4): 211–215. doi:10.1080/03009740310003695.

Hatheway CL (1990) Toxigenic clostridia. Clinical Microbiology Reviews 3(1): 66–98.

Hollander D (1999) Intestinal permeability, leaky gut, and intestinal disorders. Current Gastroenterology Reports 1(5): 410–416. doi:10.1007/s11894-999-0023-5.

Hooper LV and Gordon JI (2001) Commensal host-bacterial relationships in the gut. Science 292(5519): 1115–1118. doi:0.1126/science.1058709.

Hooper LV, Littman DR and Macpherson AJ (2012) Interactions between the microbiota and the immune system. Science 336(6086): 1268–1273. doi:0.1126/science.1223490.

Hsiao EY, McBride SW, Hsien S, Sharon G, Hyde ER, McCue T, Codelli JA, Chow J, Reisman SE, Petrosino JF, Patterson PH and Mazmanian SK (2013) Microbiota modulate behavioral and physiological abnormalities associated with neurodevelopmental disorders. Cell 155(7): 1451–1463. doi:10.1016/j.cell.2013.11.024.

Jackson ML, Butt H, Ball M, Lewis DP and Bruck D (2015) Sleep quality and the treatment of intestinal microbiota imbalance in Chronic Fatigue Syndrome: A pilot study. Sleep Science 8(3): 124–133. doi:http://dx.doi.org/10.1016/j.slsci.2015.10.001.

Kang D-W, Park JG, Ilhan ZE, Wallstrom G, LaBaer J, Adams JB and Krajmalnik-Brown R (2013) Reduced incidence of Prevotella and other fermenters in intestinal microflora of autistic children. PloS One 8(7): e68322. doi:10.1371/journal.pone.0068322.

Kanner L (1943) Autistic disturbances of affective contact. Nervous Child 2: 217–250.

Kohane IS, McMurry A, Weber G, MacFadden D, Rappaport L, Kunkel L, Bickel J, Wattanasin N, Spence S, Murphy S and Churchill S (2012) The co-morbidity burden of children and young adults with autism spectrum disorders. PloS One 7(4): e33224. doi:10.1371/journal.pone.0033224.

Leskovec TJ, Rowles BM and Findling RL (2008) Pharmacological treatment options for autism spectrum disorders in children and adolescents. Harvard Review of Psychiatry 16(2): 97–112. doi:10.1080/10673220802075852.

Li Q, Han Y, Dy ABC and Hagerman RJ (2017) The gut microbiota and autism spectrum disorders. Frontiers in Cellular Neuroscience 11. doi:10.3389/fncel.2017.00120.

Logan A, Venket A and Irani D (2003) Chronic fatigue syndrome: lactic acid bacteria may be of therapeutic value. Medical Hypotheses 60(6): 915–923. doi:10.1016/S0306-9877(03)00096-3.

Masi A, Lampit A, DeMayo M, Glozier N, Hickie I and Guastella A (2017) A comprehensive systematic review and meta-analysis of pharmacological and dietary supplement interventions in paediatric autism: moderators of treatment response and recommendations for future research. Psychological Medicine 47(7): 1323–1334. doi:10.1017/S0033291716003457.

Matson JL and Shoemaker M (2009) Intellectual disability and its relationship to autism spectrum disorders. Research in Developmental Disabilities 30(6): 1107–1114. doi:10.1016/j.ridd.2009.06.003.

Nikolov RN, Bearss KE, Lettinga J, Erickson C, Rodowski M, Aman MG, McCraken JT, McDougle CJ, Tierney E, Vitiello B, Arnold LE, Shah B, Posey DJ, Ritz L and Scahill L (2009) Gastrointestinal symptoms in a sample of children with pervasive developmental disorders. Journal of Autism and Developmental Disorders 39(3): 405–413. doi:10.1007/s10803-008-0637-8.

Parracho HM, Bingham MO, Gibson GR and McCartney AL (2005) Differences between the gut microflora of children with autistic spectrum disorders and that of healthy children. Journal of Medical Microbiology 54(10): 987–991. doi:10.1099/jmm.0.46101-0.

Penders J, Thijs C, van den Brandt PA, Kummeling I, Snijders B, Stelma F, van Ree R and Stobberingh EE (2007) Gut microbiota composition and development of atopic manifestations in infancy: the KOALA Birth Cohort Study. Gut 56(5): 661–667. doi:10.1136/gut.2006.100164.

Perry A, Flanagan HE, Geier JD and Freeman NL (2009) Brief report: The vineland adaptive behavior scales in young children with autism spectrum disorders at different cognitive levels. Journal of Autism and Developmental Disorders 39(7): 1066–1078. doi:10.1007/s10803-009-0704-9.

Rao AV, Bested AC, Beaulne TM, Katzman MA, Iorio C, Berardi JM and Logan AC (2009) A randomized, double-blind, placebo-controlled pilot study of a probiotic in emotional symptoms of chronic fatigue syndrome. Gut Pathogens 1(1): 6. doi:10.1186/1757-4749-1-6.

Sandler RH, Finegold SM, Bolte ER, Buchanan CP, Maxwell AP, Väisänen ML, Nelson MN and Wexler HM (2000) Short-term benefit from oral vancomycin treatment of regressive-onset autism. Journal of Child Neurology 15(7): 429–435.

Seida JK, Ospina MB, Karkhaneh M, Hartling L, Smith V and Clark B (2009) Systematic reviews of psychosocial interventions for autism: an umbrella review. Developmental Medicine and Child Neurology 51(2): 95–104. doi:10.1111/j.1469-8749.2008.03211.x.

Sekirov I, Russell SL, Antunes LCM and Finlay BB (2010) Gut microbiota in health and disease. Physiological Reviews 90(3): 859–904. doi:10.1152/physrev.00045.2009.

Simonoff E, Pickles A, Charman T, Chandler S, Loucas T and Baird G (2008) Psychiatric disorders in children with autism spectrum disorders: prevalence, comorbidity, and associated factors in a population-derived sample. Journal of the American Academy of Child and Adolescent Psychiatry 47(8): 921–929. doi:0.1097/CHI.0b013e318179964f.

Song Y, Liu C and Finegold SM (2004) Real-time PCR quantitation of clostridia in feces of autistic children. Applied and Environmental Microbiology 70(11): 6459–6465. doi:10.1128/AEM.70.11.6459-6465.2004.

Stigler KA, Sweeten TL, Posey DJ and McDougle CJ (2009) Autism and immune factors: A comprehensive review. Research in Autism Spectrum Disorders 3(4): 840–860. doi:http://dx.doi.org/10.1016/j.rasd.2009.01.007.

Sullivan Å, Nord CE and Evengård B (2009) Effect of supplement with lactic-acid producing bacteria on fatigue and physical activity in patients with chronic fatigue syndrome. Nutrition Journal 8(1): 4. doi:10.1186/1475-2891-8-4.

Taur Y, Xavier JB, Lipuma L, Ubeda C, Goldberg J, Gobourne A, LeeYJ, Dubin KA, Socci ND, Viale A, Perales MA, Jeng PR, van denBrink MR and Pamer EG (2012) Intestinal domination and the risk of bacteremia in patients undergoing allogeneic hematopoietic stem cell transplantation. Clinical Infectious Diseases 55(7): 905–914. doi:10.1093/cid/cis580.

Wang L, Christophersen CT, Sorich MJ, Gerber JP, Angley MT and Conlon MA (2013) Increased abundance of *Sutterella* spp. and Ruminococcus torques in feces of children with autism spectrum disorder. Molecular Autism 4(1): 42. doi:0.1186/2040-2392-4-42.

Williams BL, Hornig M, Buie T, Bauman ML, Paik MC, Wick I, Bennett A, Jabado O, Hirschberg DL and Lipkin WI (2011) Impaired carbohydrate digestion and transport and mucosal dysbiosis in the intestines of children with autism and gastrointestinal disturbances. PloS One 6(9): e24585. doi:10.1371/journal.pone.0024585.

Wing L (1988) The continuum of autistic characteristics. Diagnosis and Assessment in Autism (pp. 91–110): Springer.

Chapter 14

The Probiotics Evidence-base
Improving Quality through Innovation in Research Methodologies

Colin R Martin[1],* and *Derek Larkin*[2]

INTRODUCTION

The probiotics evidence-base represents a developing area of research endeavour, characterised by a myriad of approaches to research design from single-case to randomised controlled trials. A critical area of consideration as research in this area develops and matures is to reflect on both the quality of the contemporary evidence base and also the development of facilitative approaches to the enhancement of high quality probiotics research activity in the future. It is clear that the contemporary probiotics evidence base is incredibly diffuse, both in terms of quality of studies and approach to methodologies. There are many reasons for this. Firstly, the area of probiotics research and the application of research findings is incredibly broad, thus unlike a classical clinical area defined by diagnostic signs and symptoms, research within the probiotics field is characterised by breadth, especially in relation to methodological approaches taken and also in terms of application. This presents a potential dilemma within the field since there is the danger of presenting a 'solution in need of a problem' since in the traditional sense, probiotic research activity is geared toward well-being rather than rising from a distinct and unitary model of pathology that is accompanied by an etiological architecture with clearly defined diagnostic and prognostic architecture. Secondly, probiotics research in terms of

[1] Faculty of Society and Health, Buckinghamshire New University, Uxbridge Campus, 106 Oxford Road, Uxbridge, Middlesex, UB8 1NA, UK.
[2] Edge Hill University, St Helens Road, Ormsirk, Lancashire, L39 4QP.
* Corresponding author

its current stage of evolution can be considered at three fundamental strands, these being; (i) basic science, (ii) theory-building and (iii) efficacy of intervention. Given the breadth of activity and the scope of the strands outlined, it can be no surprise that apart from a small number of 'hotspots', probiotics research activity is spread incredibly thinly, a situation which may impact deleteriously on the quality of studies conducted and also the penetration of findings into the mainstream human sciences and biochemistry research literature. Thirdly, and invariably a contemporary endpoint influenced significantly by points one and two, is difficulty in replicating findings from studies that have been conducted, included those which furnish compelling evidence that could potentially contribute to the knowledge base. Interestingly, this issue of problems with replication is by no means not exclusive to probiotics research and indeed, has recently been raised as a critical and fundamental issue for the behavioural and psychological sciences, for example, Fisher et al. (1989). However, given the considerable and established evidence-base of the behavioural sciences accrued over at least the past one hundred years and the finding that problems of replication represents a topical blight on activity within that field, the ramification of the replication issue to the area of probiotics can be argued to be somewhat magnified, given the relative recent emergence of probiotics research as a scientific activity.

Finally, consideration must be given to the context of research specifically within the probiotics field and with respect to other disciplines, in particular basis biological sciences and applied health research, in terms of the minimum acceptable standards that would be anticipated for a good research output, for example a peer-reviewed journal with an impact factor. To demonstrate equity with other disciplines, particularly those with an applied health focus, probiotics research will necessarily need to demonstrate methodological rigour and robustness and replicability and to do this consistently. Methodological rigour and replicability represent the foundation stones of good clinical science, complimented by sound theoretical underpinnings and an incremental approach to knowledge generation and affirmation (Hood, 2009; Madeo et al., 1998; Reynolds et al., 2011; Thompson and Martin, 2017; Ulrich et al., 2008). It is therefore completely plausible and reasonable to advocate equity between probiotics research activity and other health research activity on the basis of methodological transparency, robustness and replicability. Across the field of probiotics research, this, for the reasons highlighted above, represents a significant shortcoming in need of redress. A critical question then, is what can be done to improve quality and impact of studies?

Research Design Considerations

Detailed in Figure 1 is the traditional hierarchy of evidence that is often used to define quality in terms of biomedical research. The persistence of the model is largely circumscribed by the acknowledgement that quality of evidence is bound by specific types of research design.

It can be seen in Figure 1 at the very lowest of credible evidence is the 'expert opinion and editorials'. Somewhat of a surprise for some experts surely is the low comparative weighting given to these forms of evidence. However, this should not come as too much of a surprise given that expert opinions are merely that, opinions

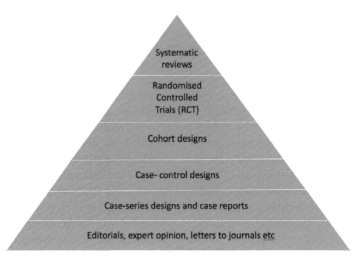

Figure 1 The pyramid of evidence ranging from low to high quality evidence at the peak.

based on available and often 'cherry-picked' evidence. The nature of opinion means that these are unlikely to be free from bias and within the context of an evidence vacuum, the bias is likely to be attenuated. There are many good examples of this in relative recent history in the natural evolution of the evidence base of controversial clinical presentations. A good example is the chronic fatigue syndrome/myalgic encephalopathy (CFS/ME). It is notable that the CFS/ME has been a hotly contested disorder in terms of aetiology over the past twenty plus years with competing disciplines arguing that the disorder is of either psychiatric or of physiological, for example, post-infective, immunological, etc., origin. Importantly, the weight of evidence regarding CFS/ME has transitioned from a psychiatric presentation to a clinical entity of likely physiological origin (Blundell et al., 2015; Gerwyn and Maes, 2017; Larkin and Martin, 2017; Mallet et al., 2016; Wallis et al., 2017). Prior to the accrual of evidence that CFS/ME has legitimate physiological underlying mechanisms and the development of coherent physiologically-bounded aetiological mechanisms, 'expert opinion' and 'editorials' were often very disparaging about the disorder and indeed the unfortunate patients experiencing the disorder. Thus, the evidence vacuum attenuated the 'expert opinions' and the content of editorials in an often negative, unhelpful and uninformed manner. Given the controversy that surrounds the underlying biological modus operandi of probiotics and the potential application of findings to improvement and enhancement of well-being, it is likely that evidence informed by expert opinion and editorials within the field will be susceptible to the same biases and negatively as has been seen within the CFS/ME field. This is also true of the expert opinion and editorials of 'ideological zealots' who may be very positive about the role of probiotics but do not characterise their articulations within robust clinical or experimental contexts. Rightly then, the expert opinion and editorial remains at the low end of the spectrum when considering the veracity of probiotics research.

Case series and case reports represent a more robust layer of evidence than editorials and expert opinion, however, their credibility can be challenged by wide variation between cases making plausible inferences difficult in terms of probiotic action and effect. Related also to the points raised earlier about the diversity and breadth of probiotic research, reach and potential application, the value of case-control studies is limited essentially by the agreement and definition of an outcome. Generally, outcomes are not circumscribed within the probiotics field by say, exposure to a pathogen and then an appraisal to an outcome that can be compared to a control participant. This represents for probiotics a divergence between the traditional medical paradigm of exposure, course, treatment and outcome for which probiotics does not have a comparative equivalent. Therefore, case-control approaches may not be the most appropriate approach to the generation of high quality evidence of probiotic action. Cohort study designs, in contrast, may be more valuable in terms of understanding potential applications of probiotics if for example, an analogue of probiotic action can be identified in one group, in terms of an 'exposure' and not in another group 'non-exposed', in order to facilitate comparison and gain insights into potential group differences. The longitudinal nature of this design type and the current level of maturity of probiotics research activity, likely raises limitations for this type of design also, though potentially it is promising as the mechanistic underpinnings of action of probiotics becomes more understood.

The 'gold standard' approach that may, at a stroke, enhance the credibility, standing and reach of probiotics research is the utilisation of the randomised controlled trial (RCT) design. The RCT is the standard and established research paradigm used within clinical trials, specifically those around demonstrating the efficacy of a new drug against either treatment as usual (TAU) or a placebo group. The strengths of the RCT is experimental robustness, an artefact of random allocation of participants to either the 'treatment' or 'control' group, and inherent methodological procedures to reduce confounding of the study such as 'double-blinding', thus neither the participant or the researcher knows which group the participant has been allocated to until the double-blind is 'broken'. It is important to acknowledge that the RCT design is not only the preserve of the pharmaceutical industry, but due to its methodological rigour and applicability, this design type has also been utilised in a broad range of health-related outcome activity, including that of assessing behavioural outcomes and interventions (Rosenthal et al., 2014; Tylee et al., 2012). It should therefore be incumbent on probiotics researchers to carefully consider whether an RCT design is both feasible and realisable for an evaluative study given this design's inherent robustness and proximity to the zenith of best practice for evidence accrual as a design type. Bringing together the findings of the best quality studies is the preserve of the systematic review, hence the pre-eminence given to these reviews at the top of the evidence pyramid. However, as is clear from the above, in order to conduct a systematic review, there needs to be studies available which are both comparable and of adequate quality to be incorporated into the systematic review process.

Issues of Sample Size

Irrespective of the type of design chosen for quantitative studies examining the influence, role, efficacy or mode of action of probiotics, it is noticeable in the literature that there exists large variability in the sample size of studies. Many studies do not report a sample size calculation and in combination with a small sample it is often difficult to determine if any lack of effect is due to that, that there is no true effect, or that the study may itself be underpowered, thus there is an effect but that it is not detected through null-hypothesis significance testing (NHST). Confusion over sample size is magnified by the common occurrence in the biological science field of often having a small sample size due to restrictions in data collection opportunities, resources, etc., but against a backdrop of an anticipated large effect size. Thus, in this context, a large effect size, even a small sample study may demonstrate statistical significance. However, in the probiotics field, the notion of large effects sizes might not readily extrapolate. Rather than conduct an underpowered study, we would advocate, where possible and where feasible, and in the absence of any prior data available to inform an appropriate sample size, to conduct a *pilot* study with the goal of not only determining potential issues with the study design but also with the *specific* goal of estimating, from data, the effect size of any probiotic intervention and then based on conventional criteria of power and alpha, calculate a sample size that is likely to give rise to a statistically significant impact of the intervention.

It may be surprising for readers to be aware that many probiotic studies are published as *main* studies with sample sizes that fall below those of a *pilot* study if one is to use the example of a simple between-groups study with criterion alpha = 0.05, power ($1-\beta$) of 0.8 and the specification of a large effect size of 0.8 (Cohen, 1977), two-tailed. This gives a total sample size of N = 52 (N = 26 per group). Importantly, even if predicting a large effect, which as mentioned is often unlikely in probiotics research contexts, the specification of a minimum N for the pilot study will enable the effect size to be calculated and an appropriate sample size for the *main* study to be effectively and efficiently calculated. Consistent with a view of parsimony, we would suggest that in circumstances where it is feasible and within the context of the design type specified (between-groups), a minimum sample size of N = 52 is highly desirable. Taking this approach, the probiotics researcher will be able to conduct a robust pilot study, calculate effect sizes and as an additional benefit, have the reassurance that if there is generally a large effect, it will not only be detected by the pilot study, but that there would be no need for a larger sample size, in effect, in this context the pilot study becomes the main study. Using the above design paradigm but calculating a medium effect of 0.5 a sample size of N = 128 (N = 64 per group) would be required in order to detect a statistically significant difference. Arguing further that, and within the context of the classical medical paradigm that even small effects are clinically relevant, thus specifying an effect size of 0.2, a total sample size of N = 788 is required (N = 394 per group) in order to be likely to detect a statistically significant difference. It is thus apparent that sample size is fundamental to not only the outcome but also the interpretation of probiotic studies and should be an important consideration at the outset.

Given that underpowered studies abound, differentiating between no effect and an occluded true effect becomes extremely difficult. Interestingly, this also has ramifications for the degree and type of detail reported in summaries of probiotic studies of this type of design, or indeed any that are quantitatively based and evaluated by inferential statistics. If one were to review say, for example, a small N (potentially underpowered) probiotics study that revealed no statistically significant difference of the intervention but adequately reported key statistical information, the reader would indeed be able to calculate both the effect size and sample size needed to be likely to find a statistically significant difference. This therefore renders additional value in studies which look promising, evaluate legitimate probiotic hypotheses but fail to detect significant influence of the intervention. Couched within this rubric, these 'non-significant' studies can provide useful pilot data to other researchers in determining sample size for an adequately powered replication study, but only if group means and standard deviations are reported in the published paper. The reporting of confidence intervals is also encouraged to give additional certainty/clarify uncertainty of estimated parameters. Again, confidence intervals are often absent from the published probiotic studies irrespective of whether statistically significant effects are observed or not.

Structural Equation Modelling

The use of structural equation modelling (SEM) has become increasingly used in the behavioural sciences to evaluate complex models of association that go beyond correlational and simple regression models, for example, Nelson et al. (2008) and Cheung and Cheung (2016). The value of SEM approaches has yet to be realised within the probiotics literature to date and yet offers a great deal of promise in looking at plausible and even complex accounts of the potential relationship/s between probiotics and a range of physiological and behavioural dimensions. Importantly, the conceptual nomenclature of SEM is to evaluate a *theoretically coherent* model. Using this framework, if the model fits the data, then the model itself is assumed to be robustly and statistically convincing. Though statistically complex, SEM is fundamentally based on regression and correlation and as such, allows a great deal of dexterity in the range of models that can be tested, the main tenet being that the models themselves have a legitimate theoretical underpinning to inform the structural model to be evaluated. Using an example, a structural model could be evaluated that looks at the relationship between a biochemical index of probiotic activity and a mental health indices, for example level of depression. Should both indices be measured on at least a polytomous/ordered categorical level of measurement they can be conceptualised within a structural equation model *with* other theoretically related parameters, for example anxiety, frequency of antibiotic use, etc., and the relationships between all parameters *and interactions* modelled. Nominal data can also be incorporated into the models for evaluation for example, in a similar way to a categorical outcome variable within a logistic regression. The plausibility of the models to be tested is essential in that they must be rooted in theoretical coherence, however, what is important is that the model and by definition the relationships can be theoretically tested. There is little doubt that SEM, as a sophisticated statistical approach offers an important opportunity to probiotics researchers to evaluate theoretically informed models and establish relationships between key variables critical to the models themselves. Thus, SEM offers a robust statistical 'glue' to bind together anticipated relationships between diverse variables and assess them statistically, robustly and pragmatically. Though, as mentioned, seldom utilised within the probiotics field to date, the opportunities and insights that are potentially afforded by the evaluation of probiotic SEM are ripe for exploitation. The software to conduct such SEM analysis is now generally available and there are sufficient statisticians competent in the use of SEM to offer help, support and collaboration with such potential studies. A pertinent reflection is that given the availability of such statistical techniques and the resources to incorporate them into more sophisticated NHST it remains incumbent on the probiotics researcher themselves to generate the models that are then systematically evaluated by SEM. It is therefore hoped that the availability of such techniques offers the impetus to facilitate expression of conceptual ideas that may have previously inhabited just the researcher's individual cognitive and mental space and be evaluated within the tacit model.

Conclusion

This chapter has looked at a number of methodological challenges and indeed opportunities that more generally relate to the conduct of high quality empirical research but are also of especial pertinence and relevance to the probiotics researcher. An essential caveat to this chapter is that the focus has been invariably focused on quantitative approaches. We recognise that innovation in qualitative approaches is also of value in probiotics research, particularly from the patient experience perspective and certainly within that context, the notion of developing probiotic research paradigms that incorporate mixed-methods (Campbell et al., 2017; Dahan-Oliel et al., 2016; Guillaumie et al., 2017; Pezaro et al., 2017) approaches, is also to be encouraged. Given the shortcomings that have been identified in current approaches to research rigour in the probiotics research field, the adoption or incorporation of qualitative and indeed mixed-methods approaches at this stage of maturity of the probiotics research movement may seem to be an 'ask' too far. However, we would argue that this is not the case at all, simply that the pace of research in the probiotics field is governed by multifactorial elements and that the area itself is ripe for innovation with the use of some of the approaches outlined, recognising that these approaches themselves, for example, SEM, represent relatively recently developed innovations of great potential application to the probiotics research endeavour.

References

Blundell S, Ray KK, Buckland M and White PD (2015) Chronic fatigue syndrome and circulating cytokines: A systematic review. Brain, Behavior, and Immunity 50: 186–195. doi:10.1016/j.bbi.2015.07.004.

Campbell DJ, Tam-Tham H, Dhaliwal KK, Manns BJ, Hemmelgarn BR, Sanmartin C and King-Shier K (2017) Use of mixed methods research in research on coronary artery disease, diabetes mellitus, and hypertension: a scoping review. Circulation: Cardiovascular Quality and Outcomes 10(1). doi:10.1161/CIRCOUTCOMES.116.003310.

Cheung MW and Cheung SF (2016) Random-effects models for meta-analytic structural equation modeling: review, issues, and illustrations. Res Synth Methods 7(2): 140–155. doi:10.1002/jrsm.1166.

Cohen J (1977) Statistical Power Analysis for the Behavioral Sciences. London: Academic Press.

Dahan-Oliel N, Oliel S, Tsimicalis A, Montpetit K, Rauch F and Dogba MJ (2016) Quality of life in osteogenesis imperfecta: A mixed-methods systematic review. American Journal of Medical Genetics. Part A 170A(1): 62–76. doi:10.1002/ajmg.a.37377.

Fisher DG, Anglin MD, Weisman CP and Pulliam L (1989) Replication problems of substance abuser MMPI cluster types. Multivariate Behav Res 24(3): 335–352. doi:10.1207/s15327906mbr2403_4.

Gerwyn M and Maes M (2017) Mechanisms explaining muscle fatigue and muscle pain in patients with myalgic encephalomyelitis/chronic fatigue syndrome (ME/CFS): a review of recent findings. Current Rheumatology Reports 19(1): 1. doi:10.1007/s11926-017-0628-x.

Guillaumie L, Boiral O and Champagne J (2017) A mixed-methods systematic review of the effects of mindfulness on nurses. Journal of Advanced Nursing 73(5): 1017–1034. doi:10.1111/jan.13176.

Hood MN (2009) A review of cohort study design for cardiovascular nursing research. Journal of Cardiovascular Nursing 24(6): E1–9. doi:10.1097/JCN.0b013e3181ada743.

Larkin D and Martin CR (2017) The interface between chronic fatigue syndrome and depression: A psychobiological and neurophysiological conundrum. Neurophysiologie Clinique 47(2): 123–129. doi:10.1016/j.neucli.2017.01.012.

Madeo M, Martin CR, Turner C, Kirkby V and Thompson DR (1998) A randomized trial comparing Arglaes (a transparent dressing containing silver ions) to Tegaderm (a transparent polyurethane dressing) for dressing peripheral arterial catheters and central vascular catheters. Intensive and Critical Care Nursing 14(4): 187–191.

Mallet M, King E and White PD (2016) A UK based review of recommendations regarding the management of chronic fatigue syndrome. Journal of Psychosomatic Research 88: 33–35. doi:10.1016/j.jpsychores.2016.07.008.

Nelson TD, Aylward BS and Steele RG (2008) Structural equation modeling in pediatric psychology: overview and review of applications. Journal of Pediatric Psychology 33(7): 679–687. doi:10.1093/jpepsy/jsm107.

Pezaro S, Clyne W and Fulton EA (2017) A systematic mixed-methods review of interventions, outcomes and experiences for midwives and student midwives in work-related psychological distress. Midwifery 50: 163–173. doi:10.1016/j.midw.2017.04.003.

Reynolds RF, Lem JA, Gatto NM and Eng SM (2011) Is the large simple trial design used for comparative, post-approval safety research? A review of a clinical trials registry and the published literature. Drug Safety 34(10): 799–820. doi:10.2165/11593820-000000000-00000.

Rosenthal EL, Balcazar HG, De Heer HD, Wise S, Flores L and Aguirre M (2014) Critical reflections on the role of CBPR within an RCT community health worker prevention intervention. Journal of Ambulatory Care Management 37(3): 241–249. doi:10.1097/JAC.0000000000000010.

Thompson DR and Martin CR (2017) Bayes' theorem and its application to cardiovascular nursing. European Journal of Cardiovascular Nursing, 1474515117712317. doi:10.1177/1474515117712317.

Tylee A, Haddad M, Barley E, Ashworth M, Brown J, Chambers J, Farmer A, Fortune Z, Lawton R, Leese M, Mann A, McCrone P, Murray J, Pariante C, Phillips R, Rose D, Rowland G, Sabes-Figuera R, Smith A and Walters P (2012) A pilot randomised controlled trial of personalised care for depressed patients with symptomatic coronary heart disease in South London general practices: the UPBEAT-UK RCT protocol and recruitment. BMC Psychiatry 12: 58. doi:10.1186/1471-244X-12-58 PMCID:PMC3437191.

Ulrich RS, Zimring C, Zhu X, DuBose J, Seo HB, Choi YS, Quan X and Joseph A (2008) A review of the research literature on evidence-based healthcare design. HERD 1(3): 61–125.

Wallis A, Ball M, McKechnie S, Butt H, Lewis DP and Bruck D (2017) Examining clinical similarities between myalgic encephalomyelitis/chronic fatigue syndrome and D-lactic acidosis: a systematic review. Journal of Translational Medicine 15(1): 129. doi:10.1186/s12967-017-1229-1 PMCID:PMC5463382.

Index

Editors Biography

Colin R Martin is Professor of Mental Health at Buckinghamshire New University, Middlesex, UK. He is a Registered Nurse, Chartered Health Psychologist and a Chartered Scientist. He has published or has in press well over 250 research papers and book chapters. He is a keen book author and editor having written and/or edited several books all of which reflect his diverse academic and clinical interests that examine in-depth, the interface between mental health and physical health. These outputs include the *Handbook of Behavior, Food and Nutrition (2011), Perinatal Mental Health: A Clinical Guide (2012), Nanomedicine and the Nervous System (2012), and the major reference works Comprehensive Guide to Autism (2014), Diet and Nutrition in Dementia and Cognitive Decline (2015), Comprehensive Guide to Post-Traumatic Stress Disorder (2016)* and *Metabolism and Pathophysiology of Bariatric Surgery: Nutrition, Procedures, Outcomes and Adverse Effects (2017).*

Dr Derek Larkin is a Senior Lecturer at Edge Hill University, having previously conducted research at The University of Manchester, University of Hull, and Keele University. He is a Chartered Psychologist, and an Associate Fellow at the British Psychological Society. Derek's research focus within neuroscience and psychology has lead him to conduct clinical research specifically in how food shapes our world—from consuming too little to consuming too much, and the psychiatric hurdles that we all face when making food choices.

Printed and bound by CPI Group (UK) Ltd, Croydon, CR0 4YY

01/11/2024

01782623-0017